The Official Guide to the Longest Wilderness Footpath in Texas

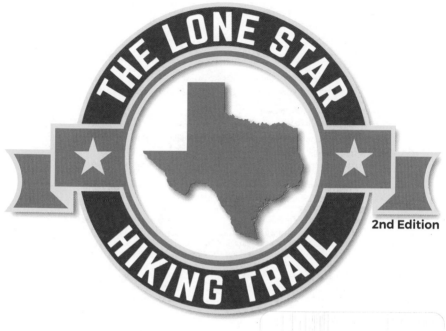

2nd Edition

T0160667

Karen Borski Somers

WILDERNESS PRESS . . . *on the trail since 1967*

The Lone Star Hiking Trail: The Official Guide to the Longest Wilderness Footpath in Texas

Copyright © 2009 and 2020 by Karen Borski Somers
All rights reserved
Printed in China
Published by Wilderness Press
Distributed by Publishers Group West
Second edition, second printing 2021

Editor: Ritchey Halphen
Photos: Karen Borski Somers, except as noted
Maps: Andy Somers, Karen Borski Somers, and Steve Jones
Cover design: Scott McGrew
Text design: Jonathan Norberg and Monica Ahlman
Proofreaders: Emily C. Beaumont, Kate Johnson
Indexer: Joanne Sprott/Potomac Indexing

Library of Congress Cataloging-in-Publication Data

Names: Somers, Karen Borski, 1971–
Title: The Lone Star hiking trail : the official guide to the longest wilderness footpath in Texas /
    Karen Borski Somers.
Description: 2nd edition. | Birmingham, AL : Wilderness Press, An imprint of AdventureKEEN, [2019]
    Includes bibliographical references and index. | Summary:
"One of the hidden jewels of Texas, the Lone Star Hiking Trail (LSHT) is the only long-distance
    National Recreation Trail in the state. At 128 miles—including loop trails—it is the state's longest
    continuously marked and maintained footpath. Located in East Texas's famed Big Thicket area,
    the trail winds through the thick woodlands of Sam Houston National Forest, an ecologically
    diverse region within a few hours' drive of Houston–Galveston, Dallas–Fort Worth, Austin, and
    San Antonio." —Provided by publisher.
Identifiers: LCCN 2019020727 | ISBN 9780899978888 (pbk.) | ISBN 9780899978895 (ebk.)
Subjects: LCSH: Hiking—Texas—Lone Star Trail—Guidebooks. | Lone Star Trail (Tex.)
Classification: LCC GV199.42.T492 L667 2019 | DDC 796.5109764/243—dc23
LC record available at https://lccn.loc.gov/2019020727

🔊 WILDERNESS PRESS

An imprint of AdventureKEEN
2204 First Ave. S., Ste. 102
Birmingham, AL 35233
800-678-7006

Visit wildernesspress.com for a complete listing of our books and for ordering information. Contact us at
info@wildernesspress.com, facebook.com/wildernesspress1967, or twitter.com/wilderness1967 with questions
or comments. To find out more about who we are and what we're doing, visit blog.wildernesspress.com.

Cover photo: The Piney Woods of East Texas characterize much of the terrain along the Lone Star Hiking Trail;
photo: Tim Maddoux

Page 5: Photo courtesy of the East Texas Research Center, Steen Library, Forest History Collections, Thompson
Family Lumber Enterprises Collection, P90T:202, Stephen F. Austin State University, Nacogdoches, Texas.
Used with permission.

SAFETY NOTICE Although Wilderness Press and the author have made every attempt to ensure that
the information in this book is accurate at press time, they are not responsible for any loss, damage, injury,
or inconvenience that may occur to anyone while using this book. You are responsible for your own safety
and health while in the wilderness. The fact that a trail is described in this book does not mean that it
will be safe for you. Be aware that trail conditions can change from day to day. Always check local conditions,
know your own limitations, and consult a map.

CONTENTS

||||||||||||||||||||||||||||||||||||||||||||||||||||||||||||||||||||||||||||||||||||||||||||||||||||||||||||||||||||||||||||||||||||||||||||||||

APPENDIXES   155

ACKNOWLEDGMENTS   174

INDEX   176

ABOUT THE AUTHOR   182

THE LONE STAR HIKING TRAIL CLUB   184

DEDICATION

For June and Jo

And for all those lost to us.

May they be just ahead around the bend in the trail that we haven't yet reached.

FOREWORD

By Marcus Woolf

IT'S STRANGE TO MARCH down a trail with a measuring wheel, slowly ticking off the distance, foot by foot, watching carefully for that magic number—5,280 feet, the number of feet in a mile. Time to once again hit the reset button.

Mapping a trail and simply hiking it are two very different things. Creating a guidebook requires incredible discipline and attention to detail, and this is precisely what Karen Somers brings to *The Lone Star Hiking Trail*. As she measures each step, she notes the fine details—seasonal streams, potential camping spots, and the character of the forest, from the "junglelike" feel of a stand of dwarf palmettos to the waterfall in a "secret nook" of the trail's Magnolia Section. Accompanying her descriptive prose are helpful charts that allow hikers to quickly glance at notable waypoints that lie along the way. Karen achieves a great balance with her work, carefully weaving together crucial data and keen observations that will pique a hiker's interest. It is one thing to tell people when to turn left or right and where water sources lie; it is another to capture the sights and sounds of a place and draw the reader into the scene.

Many people take the first steps toward writing a guidebook but soon abandon the project due to the sheer effort involved. Others enjoy a few days of hiking where they jot down the various plants, animals, and natural features along the way. And more hikers have embraced the idea of marking their routes with a GPS unit. But to do these things, and more, day after day, in blazing heat, numbing cold, or relentless downpour—this is where many book projects wither.

Having written my own trail guide for the Atlanta area, I can appreciate Karen's determination in mapping the 128 miles that make up the Lone Star Hiking Trail and nearby loops. The complex nature of the project—recording information with the GPS, writing notes, taking photographs, pushing that wheel—can become a weary exercise. At some point, a person's love for a place and the desire to share it become the fuel that sustains the effort. One thing

I know from seeing this piece of work is that Karen has a special place in her heart for this path and the wild lands of her native Texas.

A project like this requires not only love but practical experience as well. Karen has thru-hiked the 2,175-mile Appalachian Trail and the 2,650-mile Pacific Crest Trail. When she and her husband, Andy, trekked along the PCT, Karen published a wonderfully descriptive blog that first introduced me to her writing ability and keen eye. That five-month journey over formidable terrain honed her mapping skills and gave her the confidence to chronicle the Lone Star Hiking Trail. Under the cool blue winter skies of Texas, she often hiked with little more than the rattle of a measuring wheel to keep her company. Having experienced the same type of journey myself, I can imagine her pausing on a quiet stretch of trail and leaning over to press the reset button, watching it roll from 5,280 feet to 0. With many more miles to go, I can picture her standing still for a moment to hear the wind in the pines. She wipes the sweat from her brow and smiles, remembering that this is not just work, but a chance to share something wonderful.

MARCUS WOOLF *has worked as an editor and writer for outdoor trade and consumer media for more than 20 years. He is the author of* Afoot & Afield Atlanta *(Wilderness Press).*

PREFACE TO THE SECOND EDITION

A LOT HAS CHANGED in the decade since I set out on a new and sometimes intimidating adventure: writing the first published guidebook to the Lone Star Hiking Trail (LSHT). The trail has changed, too, seeing more usage and notoriety in local and national trail communities, winning a struggle between users that allowed it to retain its status as foot-traffic-only, and getting plenty of TLC from volunteers who have put in countless hours to brush, repair, and mark it. In a nutshell, the LSHT is better than ever—and I hope that this guidebook is too!

When it was time for a second edition, I set out to hike the length of the LSHT again. Along with desk-based research, all new field data allowed me to overhaul this guidebook with updated trail information and enhanced maps. Taking into account the trail reroute in Section 8 (see page 115), I've updated all

Well signed and well maintained, the LSHT is ready to take you on new adventures.   Photo: Jose Rodriguez

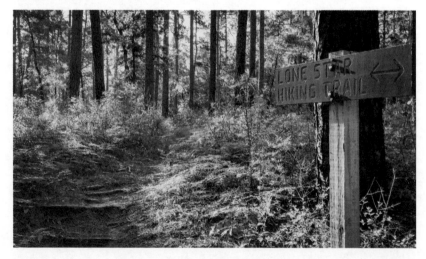

of the mileages and added mile markers to the maps. This edition also provides the locations of new primitive campsites and includes information on designated hunting-season campsites put into effect by recent U.S. Forest Service regulations.

Using on-ground hiking reports collected during the drought of 2011 by Dave Wade and the LSHT Club, I've also incorporated the club's excellent DROPS water-availability system (see page 21). Some photos have been updated, and of course I've updated the information on trail towns, shuttles, contacts, parks, and side trails. All of the step-by-step trail descriptions have been updated, noting new water sources, shortcut trails, damaged bridges, and upcoming construction plans. For consistency with other resources, the Bayou Section is now broken into two smaller sections, Tarkington and Winters Bayou. All 11 maps now include mile markers, parking-lot names, ponds, designated campsites, updated roads, and all side trails.

On my data-gathering hikes, I used a Garmin 60 CS and Garmin eTrex 10 GPS to chart the LSHT track and, ultimately, to generate the section maps. I recorded trail mileage using a mechanical measuring wheel with an error rate of approximately +/−1%. Trail descriptions and observations are based on voice notes recorded on audiotape during the hike. My original 2006 thru-hike, along with photos, is posted at trailjournals.com/lonestar.

When I was young, the Sam Houston National Forest, which sat on the shoreline just across from the Lake Conroe property that my parents owned, seemed like a vast wild place, a deep and mysterious realm. My first LSHT thru-hike in 2006 put a little dent in that notion with every road or pipeline passed, but now I can say that my perception of the forest has changed greatly. Satellite views, now so effortlessly accessed online, show the forest as a somewhat small, dark, green island of trees in a vast patchwork of civilization.

Thanks to the vision of others before us, we have a protected footpath winding for a hundred miles through this forest refuge where we can walk quietly, and alone with our thoughts if we like. Where we can take our children and show them what all of East Texas once was—where we can drink from clear streams and watch the sun set in the tall pines. More than ever before, the LSHT is a singularity and a treasure, for us and for the wild things.

One of my initial fears associated with authoring this guidebook was that, with more publicity, the LSHT would cease to be the "forgotten trail," ripe with solitude, that I first discovered back in the late 1990s. I truly thought long and hard about whether I wanted to bring more attention to the trail. But then I thought about the people living in southeast Texas who believed (just as I did once) that the best long-distance hiking trails were far away, in other states. I figured those were the people who would most love knowing that this long footpath is in their backyard—and the people who would ultimately protect it.

I took a gamble that a guidebook would be good for the LSHT, and so far this risk has paid off. The trail is in better shape, and there are more people now who respectfully walk on, care for, and protect this unique hiking trail. I hope the trail community will continue to safeguard the peace and beauty of the LSHT by keeping its entire length reserved for foot traffic only.

I strongly encourage hikers to join the LSHT Club at lonestartrail.org and the Houston Regional Group of the Sierra Club at sierraclub.org/texas /houston. Members of both groups volunteer their labor and funds to keep the LSHT marked, maintained, and open to hikers; they also plan group hikes, trail-maintenance hikes, and overnight outings, providing opportunities to support the LSHT and to meet others who enjoy hiking, backpacking, bird-watching, and nature. It's a wonderful way to stay healthy and make new friends while enjoying the trail and sharing your talents.

No matter what adventures lie in wait for you on the Lone Star Hiking Trail, I hope that this second edition of the guidebook serves you well! It has been a privilege and blessing to me to write it and to become acquainted with the people and lands of the LSHT.

Happy trails!

—*Karen Borski Somers*

FROM THE LONE STAR
HIKING TRAIL CLUB

‖‖

THE LONE STAR HIKING TRAIL (LSHT) is a jewel set in the canopied background of a dense, exotic, semitropical forest. Occasional creek bottoms and ridges offer a changing variety of trees and other plant life. There are more than 100 miles of trails accessible year-round, and more than 30 different common wild animals, including deer, wild pigs, bobcats, and coyotes. Most of the wildlife is nocturnal, but animals are occasionally seen by day hikers.

The LSHT is a window of opportunities for anyone interested in hiking. Friendships can be cultivated through club hikes, and volunteer work on the trail is a way to serve a bigger cause. Personal hiking techniques can be honed for the Continental Divide Trail or the jungles of Central America. Navigation or nighttime hiking skills can be developed. On a more personal level, hikers can simply go out, use the trails, and recharge their batteries on the weekend to return to civilization refreshed.

The Lone Star Hiking Trail Club (LSHTC) was formed in 1995 on National Trails Day and is affiliated with the American Hiking Society. Our mission is (1) to educate the public about location, use, and needs of the hiking trails of Texas, with emphasis on the LSHT, (2) to provide volunteer assistance for trail maintenance and improvement, and (3) to maintain online resources that focus on information related to hiking and maintaining trails.

Each year the members of the LSHTC lead more than 300 hikers and trail-maintenance workers on biweekly hikes and other activities, and they contribute more than 500 volunteer hours to hiker education and trail improvement.

This book is your guide to an unforgettable adventure in Sam Houston National Forest, a cosmic wonderland of nature.

—*John S. Copenhaver*
President, Lone Star Hiking Trail Club

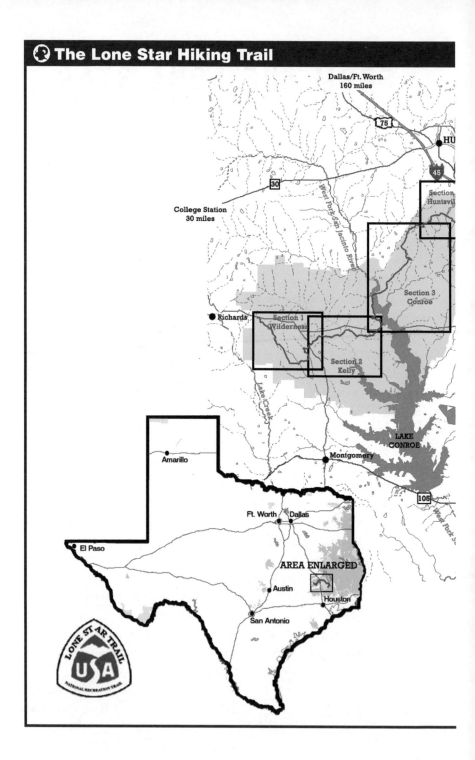

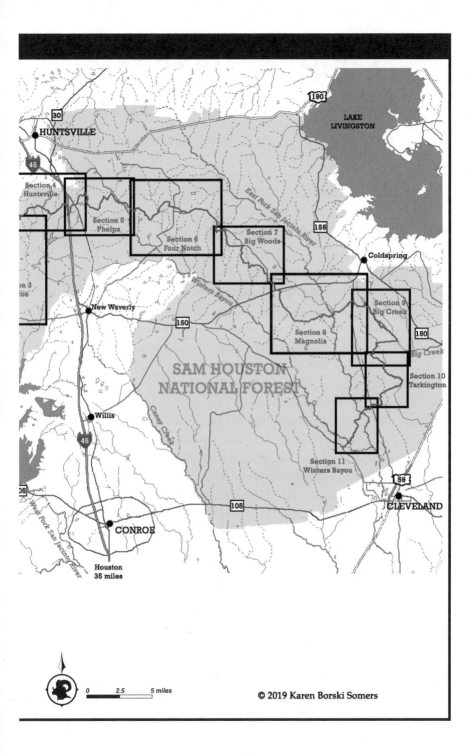

A BRIEF HISTORY
AND INTRODUCTION

||||||||||||||||||||||||||||||||||||||||||||||||||||||||||||||||||||||||||||||||||||||||||||||||||||||||||||||||||||||||||||||||||||

THE STORY OF THE LONE STAR HIKING TRAIL (LSHT) began in 1966, when a small group from the Lone Star Chapter of the Sierra Club discussed the lack of hiking trails in Texas. Orrin Bonney suggested that what was needed was a 100-mile hiking trail that would run through East Texas forests and follow old logging railroads, pipelines, and woods roads, and have places to camp every 10 miles. Other members, including Brohman Wilkin and Emil Kindschy, liked the idea and immediately began researching the feasibility. The Sierra Club approached the U.S. Forest Service (USFS), which administers Sam Houston National Forest, through which the proposed route would run.

The USFS responded positively, and in 1967 work began on the trail. Much of the trail construction was done by volunteer labor, under the auspices of the USFS, and by 1972 most of the LSHT was completed. In 1978 the last portion of the 128-mile trail (including loop trails) was finished. My own introduction to this "nature path" began in the late 1970s as a hiker on the trail. Like my predecessors and those who will walk the LSHT far into the future, I have found delight, surprise, and solitude meandering along this shaded and secluded path.

The LSHT meanders its way through shortleaf pine–post oak uplands; loblolly pine–Southern red oak–black hickory ridges and flats; white oak–Southern magnolia–loblolly pine slopes; bottomland hardwood floodplains of the East Fork of the San Jacinto River; and Winters Bayou, Caney Creek, and Little Lake Creek, which host water oak, American elm, water hickory, hackberry, swamp chestnut oak, green ash, and many other hardwood trees.

The trail offers something for hikers of every ability, from easy scenic loops that can be done in a few hours, to sections of the trail that can be hiked in a day, to weeklong backpacking trips. Walking past the picturesque shores of Lake Conroe, slipping through the bottomlands of Caney Creek, or camping in seclusion near Winters Bayou, kids, moms, dads, Scouts, naturalists, and the

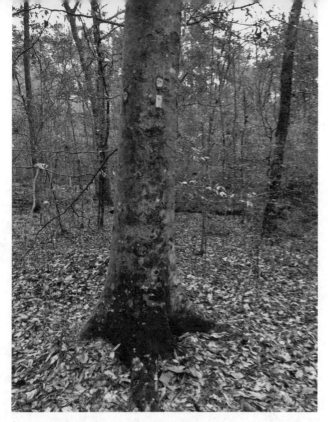

An impressive old American beech (*Fagus grandifolia*) holds Mile Marker 79 (see Section 9, page 128).

explorer and adventurer in all of us can take something from the LSHT. There are those who want to make the trail into something it is not: it's not for horses, bikes, or motorized vehicles, but it *is* for everyone with a love for wildlands, a pair of walking shoes, and the restless spirit of curiosity.

But we need to give back too. Trail maintenance is a never-ending but joyful duty and is always needed to ensure that this quiet, mysterious, footpath to solitude continues. Except for maintenance of bridges and signage by the USFS, the upkeep of the trail is performed by volunteers.

See you soon on the LSHT!

—*Brandt Mannchen*
Forest Management Issue Chair
Lone Star Chapter of the Sierra Club

CHAPTER ONE

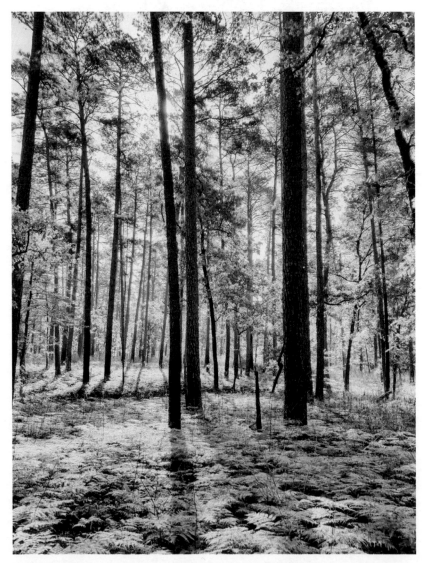

Sunlight shimmers through tall pines and illuminates the fern-blanketed forest floor. Photo: Tim Maddoux

HISTORY OF THE TRAIL

HIDDEN IN THE DEPTHS of Sam Houston National Forest, a little more than an hour from the bustle of downtown Houston, is a little-known trail where one can escape for a long, peaceful walk in the woods. This magical retreat is the Lone Star Hiking Trail (LSHT), a footpath that stretches unbroken for 96 miles through the Piney Woods of East Texas. The LSHT, part of which is designated as a National Recreation Trail, is limited to foot travel and is the longest continuously marked hiking trail in the state.

The LSHT offers hikers the chance to enjoy nature in a wilderness setting that is 70 miles north of Houston and less than a half day's drive from several other large Texas cities, including Dallas, Austin, and San Antonio. Well marked and well maintained, the trail meanders in a north-swinging arc between the small community of Richards and the town of Cleveland. Five sizeable loop trails that intersect the continuous LSHT are considered part of the trail and effectively increase its length to 128 miles. Along its course, the LSHT passes through, or near, Little Lake Creek Wilderness, Lake Conroe, Stubblefield Lake, Huntsville State Park, spring-fed Double Lake, Big Creek Scenic Area, the upper wild stretches of the East Fork of the San Jacinto River, and the pristine waterways of Winters Bayou Scenic Area.

A seemingly endless succession and variation of forests provide a paradise for tree lovers and bird-watchers. Clear-flowing, sandy-bottomed creeks, hardwood wetlands, and muddy bayous cut through gently rolling forests of pine, oak, and mixed hardwood in part of Texas's famed Big Thicket. What the LSHT lacks in wide-open views, it more than makes up for in rich, diverse woodlands and peaceful solitude. It is one of the hidden jewels of Texas.

To enjoy the trail, it's important to know a little about it: when to hike, how to get there, and what to expect. This guidebook is intended for hikers who want to explore the LSHT for any length of time or distance.

Like so many of America's great long-distance trails, the LSHT remains primarily a volunteer effort. Every year, hundreds of hours of labor are required to keep the trail clear of the very forest through which it passes. Clearing brush and fallen trees, building and repairing bridges, and repairing and replacing trail markers constitute a nonstop job undertaken primarily by volunteers from the Lone Star Hiking Trail Club, the Houston Regional Group of the Sierra Club,

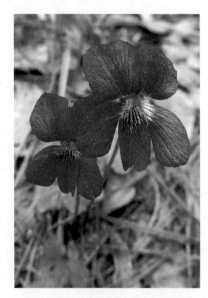

Birdstooth violets (*Viola pedata*)
commonly grace the trail in late
winter and early spring.

and the Boy Scouts of America. These organizations need ongoing funding and volunteers. As you explore the LSHT, consider becoming a trail steward by supporting these organizations or by joining a volunteer trail work crew.

Human History of the LSHT

Indigenous Peoples

The original inhabitants of southeast Texas were seminomadic hunter-gatherers who moved seasonally in search of food. During winter, they would settle in camps, or semipermanent villages, to hunt small game, deer, bears, and buffalo. In warmer months, they moved around in search of nuts, berries, fish, and roots, sometimes trading with other American Indian tribes. Some tribes also cultivated maize. Archaeological evidence indicates that American Indians inhabited what is now the Sam Houston National Forest as far back as 7,000 years ago.

The Hasinai Caddo, an offshoot tribe of the great mound-building civilization centered in the Mississippi River valley, resided between the Neches and Sabine Rivers. Because of their strong cultural roots and inland location, they tended to settle into small villages where they practiced agriculture and developed artistic clothing, wood carvings, and ceramics. The Karankawa lived nearer to the coast in small family groups, often traveling in search of food. The coastal-based subsistence living of the Karankawa, along with their unique language, kept them separate from many inland tribes.

The Atapakan-speaking tribes—the Patiri, Bidai, Deadose, and Akokisa (also spelled Orcoquisac)—lived and roamed throughout the Trinity and San Jacinto River valleys. All of these groups converged on the Big Thicket region for hunting forays and engaged in a long-distance trade network. East Texas seashells and deer skins could be traded for the furs of the northern pine marten or clay pottery from the desert southwest.

The Atapakan tribes and Karankawa succumbed to diseases introduced by early European explorers and settlers. By the mid-1800s, nearly all of the native inhabitants of southeast Texas had vanished. Only vague accounts of their cultures remain today. Some East Texas Caddo survived disease only to be driven from their native lands by the Europeans, eventually settling in Oklahoma in 1859 (where their descendants live today).

Early European Explorers

Álvar Núñez Cabeza de Vaca, a Spanish conquistador, was shipwrecked on Galveston Island on the southeast Texas coast in November 1528. Over the next four years, he lived with the American Indians of East Texas, becoming a trader and medicine man and eventually walking thousands of miles through what is now the southwestern US to Spanish outposts in Mexico. He eventually returned to Europe and published an important account of his remarkable journey through the unknown region. By the time other explorers ventured into this area almost a century later, many of the native inhabitants had already vanished, victims of disease and war. Cabeza de Vaca's account is a glimpse of East Texas before European colonization irrevocably changed the land, culture, and ecology.

The French explorer René-Robert Cavalier, Sieur de La Salle, journeyed into southeast Texas in 1687 after France laid claim to the lands of the Mississippi watershed. La Salle planned to establish outposts as he ventured northward up the Mississippi River, but he was murdered in a mutiny near Navasota, Texas, before he was able to carry out his expedition. A few years later, in 1690, the first East Texas mission was built by the Spanish for the Caddo near the settlement of Nacogdoches, an effort by Spain to gain control over the region. French influence eventually succumbed to the Spanish presence, although the French continued active trade with the Akokisa and Bidai. Eventually, in 1823, the first American pioneers settled in East Texas as part of Stephen Austin's original colony. American pioneers and frontierspeople continued to trickle into the state; they eventually formed a small militia that revolted against Mexico and won independence for Texas in 1836. As the country of Texas transitioned to US statehood in 1845, the newly arrived European residents of East Texas had already settled into the land—farming, logging, and ranching.

Logging and the Timber Industry

The logging boom peaked in East Texas starting in the 1880s and spurred the development of hundreds of mill towns. With the forests of the northern and eastern US already harvested, investors and lumberjacks flocked to the huge expanse of untapped virgin forest that covered the gently rolling lands of East Texas. By the 1920s, 18 million acres of the East Texas Piney Woods had been cut, yielding an astounding 59 billion board-feet of lumber.

Most of the mill towns and railroads that had sprung up overnight during the logging boom were quickly abandoned when the forests became depleted; the lumber companies either went bankrupt or moved westward in search of more timber. (Some of the old logging railroad beds from this era are still visible in the woods along the LSHT; in fact, the trail is actually routed on a few of them.) In 1934, the US government authorized the purchase of some of these unwanted, depleted lands in East Texas, creating Sabine, Angelina, Davy Crockett, and Sam Houston National Forests. Over the next 80 years, the U.S. Forest Service (USFS) managed the replanting and harvesting of these lands.

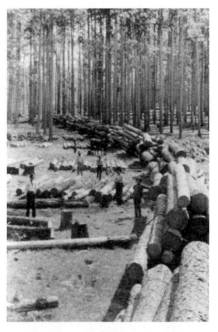

The original longleaf pines of East Texas were clear-cut and railed to mills at the turn of the 20th century.

Sam Houston National Forest

The 163,037-acre Sam Houston National Forest is contained within three Texas counties: Montgomery, San Jacinto, and Walker. The USFS is responsible for soil conservation, natural resources, and sustainable-use practices within the national forests. Their multiple-use management policy means that logging, hunting, fishing, mining, drilling, off-road vehicle use, hiking, and camping are all allowed within national forest boundaries as long as they meet the regulations of the USFS. Generally, the LSHT is routed well away from heavily used areas of the forest, but hikers should be aware that they may encounter these activities.

Although much of Sam Houston National Forest is an unbroken woodland expanse, it contains many private-land holdings, some of which force the LSHT to follow roads. Road walks can follow anything from an old dirt road to a few paved highways, taking hikers past farms, cemeteries, churches, and even contemporary neighborhoods.

Creation of the Lone Star Hiking Trail

The LSHT was conceived during a backpacking trip when a small group of Sierra Club members were camping in the Sam Houston National Forest in 1966. Lamenting that there weren't many hiking trails in the region, the hikers decided to approach the USFS to gain permission to plan and build a trail that would traverse the length of the national forest. With logistical and financial assistance from the Sierra Club and Shell Oil Company, volunteers began construction in 1967 and completed the LSHT by 1972. Long-term oversight of the trail was turned over to the USFS, but volunteers continued to maintain the trail and spent time in the late 1970s expanding the trail to its current length. Today, the LSHT is supported by the Lone Star Hiking Trail Club (LSHTC) and the Houston Regional Group of the Sierra Club, which organize volunteer maintenance efforts and oversee trail issues. Volunteers from the Boy Scouts of America also labor to keep the trail marked, bridged, and cleared.

The National Trail System Act of 1968 set the framework for the LSHT to receive federal protection; however, only the eastern 28 miles of the trail have been designated as a National Recreation Trail to date. Despite overarching regulations stating that the entire LSHT is off-limits to motorized vehicles, stock animals, wagons, and bicycles, it continues to be threatened. Its footpath-only designation is shared by only a few other trails in the US, but like many of these other trails, the LSHT continues to battle pressure from outside interests that would damage or destroy it. Without a protective buffer, other activities and interests within the national forest can damage the trail (examples include logging, road building, drilling, and fire control activities). Additionally, others want the trail opened up for use by horseback riders and mountain bikers. The Sierra Club continues to lead a

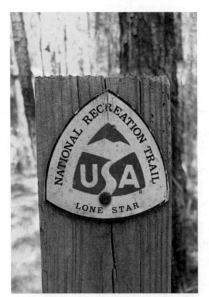

Markers along the eastern LSHT denote the 28-mile trail segment with National Recreation Trail status.

long-term fight for a protective buffer on either side of the trail, as well as an ongoing battle to maintain the LSHT's unique status as a trail preserved for foot travel only.

Natural History of the LSHT

Geology

During the Paleozoic Era, about 500 million years ago, the edge of the ancient North American continent began to rift along its southern edge. As the land subsided, a shallow inland sea formed, covering all of what is now East Texas. Subsequent periods of continental extension and compression formed basins in which thick deposits of marine salt were covered by sands and sediments, eventually forming significant oil and natural gas deposits. Later, river systems, such as the Trinity, Sabine, and Neches in East Texas, distributed more sediment on the coastal plains as they drained toward the Gulf of Mexico. The soils of East Texas are deep and rich; they are typically light-colored acidic sands, sandy loam mixed with deposits of clay (or clay-shale) and occasional mineral-rich red soils.

Plant Life

The LSHT's western terminus lies at the very edge of the great eastern deciduous forest of North America. West of the town of Richards, the land transitions from the thick Piney Woods to more-open post oak savanna and blackland prairie. Along this meeting of major biogeographic regions, complex woodlands have evolved. At first glance, the untrained eye may only see forests dominated by loblolly and shortleaf pines. If you look a little closer, however, you'll discover a unique mix of species. Sam Houston National Forest is the westernmost range of many eastern trees (such as white oak, longleaf pine, and Southern magnolia) and also home to plants that originated in drier western climates (such as prickly pear cacti and yucca). The diverse plant mosaic in this region can also be traced to the last ice age, when species from other parts of the continent moved southward.

The large terrestrial ecological region called the Piney Woods stretches across most of East Texas and into parts of Arkansas, Louisiana, and Oklahoma. It is dominated by several species of pine but is also home to a large variety of hardwood-tree species. Rather than one unbroken, homogeneous woodland, the Piney Woods comprise a tapestry of interwoven ecological environments, each supporting different species. While hiking on the LSHT, you'll see only some of the ecosystems that make up the Piney Woods and the nearby Big Thicket, an extremely biodiverse area that contains one of the highest species counts for an area of its size in the US. (Only the most remote, central part of the original Big Thicket is fully protected as a national preserve near the eastern end of the LSHT.)

Many of the region's ecological zones are easy to identify, while others may require more study using a tree guide. A few of the most common ecosystems by tree type are as follows: bottomlands composed of oak, hickory, sycamore, ash, sweetgum, alder, river birch, black willow, and maple; swamps composed of bald cypress, swamp tupelo, water hickory, and water elm; seasonally inundated flats composed of dwarf palmettos growing among a mix of hardwood trees; sloping, well-drained land comprised of American beech, Southern magnolia, and white oak; and, finally, pure stands of loblolly and shortleaf pine. A rich variety of mosses, grasses, ferns, mushrooms, and wildflowers prospers beneath the canopy of the forest. Wildflower enthusiasts can spot spring beauty, rose vervain, and Halbert-leaf rose-mallow, as well as wild orchids and sundews.

The nature of this great forest is changing; today there is more pine in proportion to hardwood. After the first wave of commercial logging denuded much of the area by the early 1900s, the fast-growing slash pine was widely planted throughout East Texas. Meanwhile, diverse bottomland ecosystems were destroyed by the creation of reservoirs. Fire was once a regular and natural force that had an integral effect on the composition of the forests, but due to human intervention, fire has been widely suppressed. The resulting monoculture pine plantations support more disease and destructive pests, such as the pine bark beetle. While the USFS has become a better steward of its lands, often prescribing burns to mimic natural conditions, it has also allowed extensive pine plantations to continue to exist in support of the timber industry.

Indeed, virtually no virgin forest remains in East Texas. During the 1970s and '80s, after the forests had somewhat recovered from their initial exploitation, clear-cutting drastically resumed. This process, along with the clearing of land for development and agriculture, has destroyed well over half of the original 5,000 square miles of habitat in East Texas that once harbored the greatest diversity of plant and wildlife in North America.

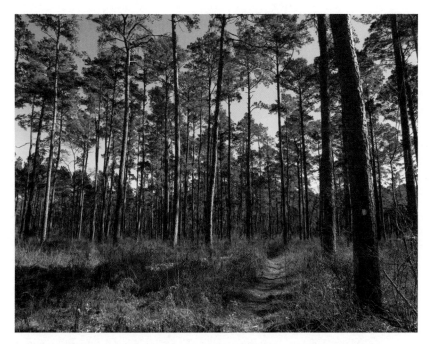

Open stands of mature pine trees, which provide a singular habitat for red-cockaded and pileated woodpeckers, are common along the western half of the LSHT.

Fortunately, LSHT hikers can still see enormous pines growing in parklike settings, miles of mature magnolias and beech, and extensive palmetto swamps. Some of these trees are more than 100 years old, yet they merely hint at what this great forest used to be. Where they're given lasting protection, East Texas's woods will continue to evolve into more complex and mature habitats resembling their former grandeur.

Animal Life

East Texas was once home to cougars, wolves, black bears, and jaguars. As Europeans began to settle the land, hunting and habitat losses took their toll, and all of these large predators gradually disappeared. Red wolves, smaller cousins to the gray wolf, were able to hang on until 1990, when the last wild individuals were trapped and removed to be placed in a captive breeding project. Coyotes and bobcats prosper and are now the largest predators remaining in East Texas. Sporadic sightings of mountain lions and black bears in East Texas have been on the rise, but no breeding populations are known to exist at the time of this writing.

Some of the species that have returned from the brink of extinction in East Texas include the river otter, beaver, bald eagle, and American alligator. The white-tailed deer and Eastern wild turkey were hunted to the point of eradication in the early 1900s and recovered only after reintroduction programs proved successful in the mid-to-late 20th century. Bison were not as fortunate—their numbers never recovered in Texas as they did in a few other areas of the US. Even today, there are mammals that face extinction in East Texas, such as the Plains spotted skunk and two bat species. Less visible endangered aquatic species found in the larger waterways of the region include the paddlefish and American eel, both of which have suffered due to reservoir construction.

Common mammals of East Texas include many well-known species of the Southeastern deciduous forest, such as the raccoon, Eastern fox squirrel, gray squirrel, and opossum. Nutrias (beaverlike rodents raised for fur) and domestic pigs are both animals that were released or that escaped into the wild and have prospered at the expense of native species. The nine-banded armadillo, which migrated northward from Mexico to the southeastern US, is the animal most likely to be seen or heard by campers. Many types of snakes and turtles, as well as amphibians, fish, and an amazing variety of insects, also inhabit the Piney Woods.

Texas is regarded as a bird-watcher's paradise. In addition to providing a comfortable climate for yearlong-resident birds, the mild winters of the Texas Gulf Coast offer refuge to scores of migratory bird species, such as the Arctic peregrine falcon. The rich and varied forest ecology of East Texas provides many differing bird habitats within a small area. The thick Piney Woods are home to the pine warbler, brown-headed nuthatch, American woodcock, barred owl, and summer tanager. Bottomlands harbor the pileated woodpecker, Carolina chickadee, and Kentucky warbler. Swamps and bayous provide homes for Swainson's warblers, wood ducks, and fish crows. Reservoirs like Lake Conroe have attracted bald eagles that spend the winter in the warm climate of East Texas.

Due to the conversion of much of the native longleaf pine–oak–palmetto forests of East Texas to pine plantation, cropland, and reservoir, many bird populations have diminished. Probably the most well-known rare bird that lives year-round in the Sam Houston National Forest is the red-cockaded woodpecker, a species that was declared endangered in 1970 and has been steadily declining over the last 15 years. These small, cardinal-sized woodpeckers are frequently spotted by observant hikers, especially near Stubblefield Lake. They require park-like stands of mature native pine trees in which to build nesting cavities; a pine habitat is now protected for these birds. The red-cockaded woodpecker has a distinctive large white cheek patch (males have a small red spot behind their eyes that give the species its name). Its unique high-pitched, squeaky call can be recognized at considerable distances.

The LSHT traverses the banks of many old, small forest ponds, some natural but most man-made, which provide an important source of water for hikers and wildlife.

CHAPTER TWO

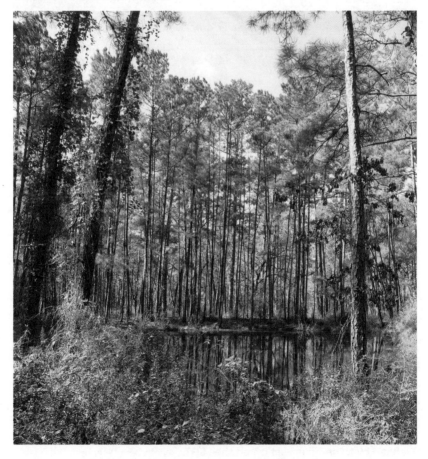

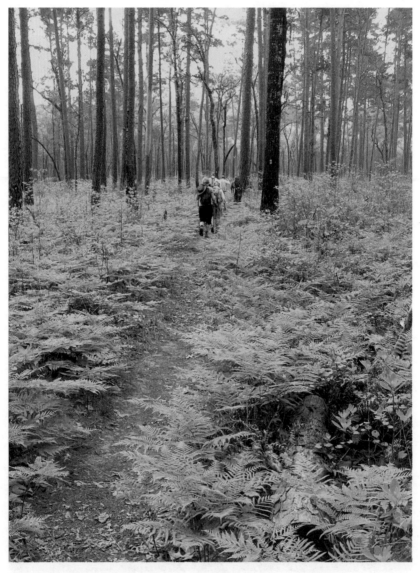

Flanked by ferns, hikers set off on the LSHT.   Photo: Cathy Murphy

HIKING
THE TRAIL

||||||||||||||||||||||||||||||||||||||||||||||||||||||||||||||||||||||||||||||||||||||||||||||||||||||||||||||||||

THE LONE STAR HIKING TRAIL (LSHT)
is the setting for adventures ranging from
short strolls to multiday backpacking trips.
Every year, a few hikers even opt to thru-
hike the LSHT, walking the whole trail in
one continuous journey. Hikers enjoy a well-
marked, nearly level trail, broken only by
a few country road walks and abounding
in backcountry camping opportunities.
Loops along the LSHT add another 32 miles
of trail to the continuous 96-mile footpath.

How to Use This Book

This guidebook focuses on the main, continuous LSHT footpath. Side trails that intersect the LSHT are noted and shown on maps but not described in detail.

For organizational purposes, the LSHT is broken into 11 sections, each roughly the length of a long day hike. Section boundaries are defined by road crossings or access points. Each section includes an overview; information on trail access, parking, water availability, access to supplies, and accommodations; a detailed trail description; a chart of GPS coordinates for major trail features; a mileage chart summarizing trail features by distance from west to east (and vice versa); and a trail map. For reference, the mileage charts are consolidated in Appendix D (page 160).

There is no right or wrong direction to hike the LSHT. This guide contains trail descriptions written from west to east only because one direction had to be chosen for the guide, and established mile markers already line the trail increasing in order from west to east. Hikers traveling from east to west will have to mentally "flip" the trail descriptions, changing left to right (and vice versa) as well as reading the trail descriptions in reverse order.

GPS coordinates, expressed in latitude and longitude, are listed for trailheads and major trail features. A key to the mileage charts follows.

MILEAGE CHART KEY

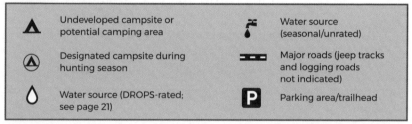

▲	Undeveloped campsite or potential camping area	🚰	Water source (seasonal/unrated)
Ⓐ	Designated campsite during hunting season	▬▬▬	Major roads (jeep tracks and logging roads not indicated)
⬥	Water source (DROPS-rated; see page 21)	P	Parking area/trailhead

Maps

The U.S. Forest Service (USFS) publishes a map of the entire Sam Houston National Forest that shows the route of the LSHT (see Appendix A, page 155, for information on ordering maps). It doesn't show as much detail as the maps in this guide, but it does provide a good overview of the area and road system surrounding the LSHT.

The detailed section maps in this book are derived from U.S. Geological Survey 7.5-minute topographic quadrangles. On each map, the LSHT is indicated by a solid line. Dotted lines show side trails that intersect the LSHT and dashed lines indicate the previous and/or next sections of the LSHT. As a general rule, larger roads are denoted by a heavier black line. Small roads (such as jeep tracks and logging roads) appear as unlabeled, dashed lines. Pipelines are dashed lines and are typically labeled. Major water features are shaded in gray.

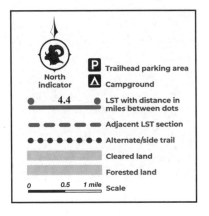

Note that not every shaded water feature is a good water source for hikers; many creeks in the area are dry most of the year. Use each section's trail description and mileage chart to help plan for your water needs.

At the time of this writing, magnetic declination—that is, the difference between magnetic north and true north—is approximately 2.5° east along the entire length of the LSHT.

The free **Maprika** mobile app for iOS and Android can used interactively to track progress during a hike; it tracks using location data when cellular service is unavailable. Within the app, search for "Lone Star" and "LSHT" to access and download a full interactive set of LSHT maps. (To prevent excessive battery drain, it's generally a good idea to keep mobile apps open and running only when needed.)

Trail and Mile Markers

The LSHT is a continuously marked footpath, meaning that a hiker walking in either direction should be able to see trail markers indicating the pathway at regular intervals, with one marker usually being in sight of the next. In addition to regular trail markers, nearly every mile of the LSHT is also marked and numbered.

LSHT **trail markers** are 2- by 4-inch unpainted aluminum plates that have been nailed to trees, posts, or poles at eye level adjacent to the trail. Double sets of markers, or tilted markers, indicate turns, trail junctions, or places where

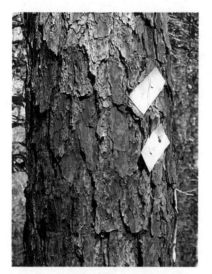

Slanted LSHT trail markers indicate a right turn ahead.

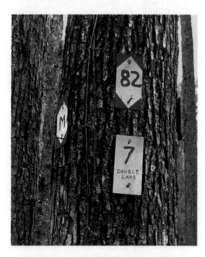

LSHT mile markers, indicating the number of miles from the western terminus, are located in trees just above eye level. Some mile markers near Double Lake also show the miles from Double Lake Recreation Area.

hikers should pay particular attention to the route. Three markers placed together indicate one of several designated primitive backcountry camping areas along the LSHT. A marker with a white stripe at its midsection indicates a junction of the main LSHT with a loop trail. Other intersecting trails are marked with colored paint or striped metal markers. Old-style LSHT markers were 3-inch metal triangles and may still exist along some parts of the trail.

In general, the LSHT is well marked and easy to follow, but there may be spots where trail markers are missing or infrequent (usually because of tree fall or vandalism). When small sections of the trail become overgrown with brush or covered with fallen leaves, look up and scan ahead for markers. If you've been walking for more than 5 minutes and you haven't seen a trail marker, you may have wandered off the LSHT. Turn around and retrace your steps to the last place where you saw a marker. Keep in mind that markers are often absent where the LSHT follows roads—this guide includes detailed directions to help you navigate road walks.

Mile markers—diamond-shaped, red-and-white metal tags—indicate each of the 96 miles of the LSHT. Mile markers are usually placed on trees just above eye level, but some are also marked with a plastic post planted in the ground. A few miles do not appear to be marked, particularly on road walks, but mile markers can be easy to overlook while you are walking and watching the trail in front of you. The mile markers are accurate except where noted in the trail descriptions. In a few places, old wooden posts with miles marked on their tops stand along the trail; these are outdated and inaccurate.

Trail Access, Parking, and Shuttle Services

The LSHT has two dozen trailhead access points where free parking is available; these trailhead parking areas are described and mapped in each section of this book. The USFS reports a low incidence of trailhead vandalism, but it's always wise to lock valuables out of sight or in the trunk of your car. If you plan to park your car at Stubblefield Lake Campground, Huntsville State Park, or Double Lake Recreation Area, notify park personnel of your plans, and expect to pay entrance/day-use fees. (*Note:* Adjacent to each of these parks is alternative trailhead parking that doesn't require a fee.)

Hikers who have flown in from out of the region or the state have limited options for getting from the airport to the trailhead. Some hikers prefer to arrange a one-way car rental; along with its usual desks at airports, **Enterprise** (855-266-9289, enterprise.com) has rental offices in Montgomery, Conroe, and Cleveland. **Greyhound** bus service (800-231-2222, greyhound.com) runs from Houston to Conroe.

For transportation from the trailheads to nearby trail towns, the options are also limited. Hitchhiking is legal as long as you don't stand on the roadway or impede traffic. Uber and Lyft are not yet widely available in the LSHT region, but **taxi service** is available in Cleveland and Conroe, with fares running about $2–$3 per mile at press time (see Appendix A). Lastly, there are individuals who offer fee-based or even free transportation to and from the trail; they can also help with staging a hiker's car at one end of the trail. Check the LSHTC's website (lonestartrail.org), Facebook page (facebook.com/groups/lonestarhikingtrail), or Twitter feed (@lone_star_trail) for the most current information on private shuttle services. In any case, trail transportation should be arranged in advance if at all possible.

Trail Conditions

The LSHT meanders through flat to gently rolling forests of varying age and type. Altitude on the LSHT is roughly between 150 and 400 feet above sea level. Hikers never ascend more than 75 feet at a time; these climbs are extremely gentle. Creeks represent the most difficult natural features to cross on the LSHT. Large creeks, rivers, and extensive wetlands are bridged, although bridges may occasionally be destroyed during floods. (*Note:* At the time of this writing, two major trail bridges are out: Stubblefield Lake Road bridge in Section 3 and the hiker bridge over the East Fork of the San Jacinto in Section 8.) Most creeks along the trail are usually dry or contain water only a few inches deep—though some have cut V-shaped ravines up to 8 feet deep that require short, steep scrambles down and up the banks.

The LSHT traverses a broad range of soil conditions, from well-drained, sandy uplands to incessantly muddy bottomlands. Hikers shouldn't have serious difficulty negotiating muddy areas, but they should expect soggy footwear on occasion. Potentially problematic areas are noted in the trail descriptions; generally, the most persistently soggy areas (standing water covering the trail after heavy rains) along the LSHT are the bottomlands around Little Lake Creek in Section 1, Caney Creek in Section 2, Winters Bayou in Section 5, Tarkington Bayou in Section 10, and Winters Bayou in Section 11. You may encounter blowdowns (fallen trees lying across the trail) and overgrown trails, but these are usually not insurmountable obstacles. Trail conditions are always subject to change, particularly after big storms. Check with Sam Houston National Forest (936-344-6205, tinyurl.com /samhoustonnationalforest) or the LSHTC for the latest conditions.

Seasons and Weather

Biting insects, extreme heat, and fewer on-trail water sources make hiking during the long East Texas summers challenging. From May through September, temperatures can reach the upper 90s, with high humidity making the heat feel well into the triple digits. If you venture onto the trail during these months, be prepared to hike at a slower pace and protect yourself from insects. Also be aware that water sources listed in this guidebook may dry up during the hottest months.

TEMPERATURE RANGES ON THE LSHT				
MONTH	AVERAGE HIGH	AVERAGE LOW	RECORD HIGH	RECORD LOW
JAN	58°F	39°F	88°F	7°F
FEB	63°F	43°F	94°F	7°F
MAR	71°F	50°F	91°F	18°F
APR	78°F	56°F	97°F	31°F
MAY	84°F	64°F	98°F	42°F
JUN	90°F	70°F	106°F	54°F
JUL	94°F	72°F	107°F	56°F
AUG	94°F	72°F	107°F	56°F
SEPT	88°F	67°F	104°F	41°F
OCT	79°F	58°F	98°F	28°F
NOV	69°F	49°F	90°F	19°F
DEC	60°F	41°F	85°F	2°F

The best seasons for hiking on the LSHT are late fall, winter, and early spring. Fall is characterized by temperature variations that are caused by intermittent cold fronts passing southeastward through the region. Cold fronts can be slow- or fast-moving and bring rain followed by rapidly falling temperatures. Winter in East Texas is generally mild, but freezing temperatures are still possible. Sam Houston National Forest receives 45 inches of rainfall per year on average; rain tends to be heaviest in the spring and fall, but droughts or periods of heavy rain can happen any time of year.

Tornadoes are most common in the spring but can also occur in summer and fall. Hurricanes give more warning of their approach. Don't venture onto the LSHT if a hurricane is moving toward the Texas Gulf Coast, and keep a close watch on the weather during the peak of hurricane season (August and September). Although the trail is located well inland, a hurricane's high winds will reach the LSHT and can spawn tornadoes. Falling limbs and trees are common in windy conditions. Creeks and rivers can quickly rise out of their banks during heavy rains.

The following is a month-by-month guide of what to expect on the trail. Average and record temperatures are found in the chart above.

January is one of the best months to be out on the trail. Deer-hunting season ends early in the month. Daytime temperatures can range from warm to cool. Expect cool nights with temperatures below freezing on the coldest nights.

February is an excellent month to be out on the LSHT. As in January, be prepared for nighttime temperatures in the 30s and 40s, with some rare nights in the 20s. Carry warm clothes, but keep a T-shirt on hand for warmer days.

March is when the trees and bugs begin to come to life again, but it's still a great time to be in the woods. Leaves begin to unfurl, honeysuckle blooms, and birds are active. Expect a few flies and mosquitoes, but mostly enjoy the butterflies. Cold nights are possible, but rare.

April is the month of Texas's famous wildflowers. The woods have fewer flowers than the roadsides, but woodland wildflowers are unique treasures compared to their cultivated roadside cousins. Temperatures are still pleasant enough to enjoy hiking before it really warms up.

May is the wettest month of the year on average. Hiking in May is a toss-up, depending on the weather and your tolerance for heat and insects. Some days are dry and beautiful, but others are a prelude to summer.

June is the first full month of summer. Flies, ticks, spiders, mosquitoes, and chiggers come out in droves, so carry insect repellent or wear long pants. Carry plenty of water, and don't overexert yourself.

July and August are terribly hot and humid. Seasonal creeks will be dry except after heavy rains. Consider sitting these months out or taking shorter hikes in the cooler hours of the day. Don't forget insect protection!

September continues to demonstrate the brutal heat of East Texas summers, but every once in a while a minor cool front brings some relief. Bugs continue to be an issue.

October is when both hiking and deer-hunting season begin. Wear fluorescent orange hunter safety gear in the woods. Ticks are still active, but you should see fewer flies and mosquitoes.

November brings increasingly better temperatures for hiking, but deer-hunting season spans the entire month, so wear hunter safety colors. Bugs diminish.

December is a good time of the year to hike, except for the continuing concern about deer-hunting season. Deciduous trees have lost their leaves by now.

Water

Access to water on the LSHT is primarily of concern for overnight hikers. Each section includes a summary of water sources along the trail, followed by a more specific account of water sources in the trail description. I have taken great care to subjectively describe the type and quality of water that I found on my hikes.

Additionally, the Lone Star Hiking Trail Club (LSHTC) provides hikers with a new water-availability system developed after the devastating droughts of 2011. The **Drought Resistance of Point Source (DROPS)** system rates the reliability of major water sources on a scale of 1–5; it does not describe the water's quality, however. The more drops, the more reliable the source.

With the club's permission, I've incorporated the DROPS system into this second edition, using the symbols below to rate all major water sources where available (some larger water sources are not rated). Check online, including at lone startrail.org, for the most current information on water conditions; the LSHTC also publishes a drought-index rating based on current conditions that can be used in conjunction with the DROPS system. Here's a quick guide to the scale:

◊◊◊◊◊	Source withstood the 2011 drought
◊◊◊◊	Source mostly withstood the 2011 drought
◊◊◊	Source could possibly dry up in typical summer heat
◊◊	Source is likely to be dry in summer
◊	Source has water only during the very wettest periods or may be stagnant

Seasonal creeks (drainages) may appear to be lush, flowing creeks after rains, but in fact they are dry most of the year and unreliable as water sources. These water sources do not carry a DROPS rating. Each section's mileage chart provides a listing of water sources, noted with either a ◊ icon (DROPS-rated) or a 🜄 icon (seasonal/unrated). *Any water source not designated with either icon should be assumed to be extremely unreliable.*

Even though I've made every effort to record and list only dependable water sources, it's possible that these sources will be dry during your hike. so always carry more water than you think you'll need. A general rule of thumb is that each hiker needs a minimum of 3 liters of water per day in cool weather (not including water for cooking). In hot weather, carry at least 1 liter of drinking water for every 3 miles.

All natural water found along the LSHT should be filtered or chemically treated to prevent illness from waterborne parasites or bacteria. Even clear, clean-looking water can harbor microscopic organisms such as *Giardia lamblia*. Potable drinking water is available near the LSHT only from taps at Stubblefield Lake Campground, Huntsville State Park, and Double Lake Recreation Area.

Rules and Regulations

The LSHT lies mostly within Sam Houston National Forest. The rules that govern hikers on the LSHT are mostly the same as those that govern any person visiting the national forest. The big exception is that *horses, bicycles, and motorized equipment of any kind are prohibited on the LSHT*—only foot travel is allowed.

No permits are required to hike the trail or use its trailhead parking lots; fees are usually required, however, if you choose to park or camp in nearby state parks or developed campgrounds.

Dogs are permitted on the LSHT, but they must be leashed and under the owner's control at all times.

Finally, remember that damaging or removing any natural feature or historical or archaeological artifact is strictly prohibited within the national forest.

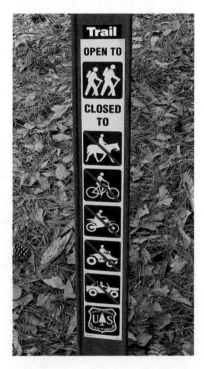

This post clearly indicates which trail uses are permitted and prohibited.

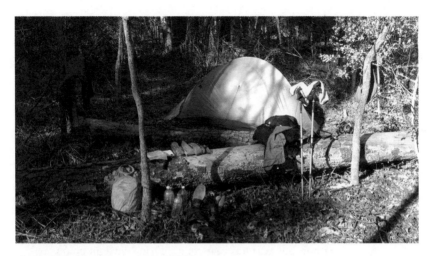

A thru-hiker's camp on the LSHT   Photo: Bill Sadd

Camping

Hikers may camp anywhere along the LSHT within Sam Houston National Forest, with the following exceptions.

The LSHT traverses one specially protected area where camping is prohibited: the **Big Creek Scenic Area** in Section 9. Camping is also prohibited inside—or within 300 feet—of any trailhead parking area.

Campers in the national forest must use specially designated sites during deer-hunting season, generally from late September to early January (exact dates vary slightly from year to year); a number of these designated sites are located along or near the LSHT. They include primitive backpacker sites, developed campgrounds, and unimproved hunting camps. The 18 designated sites are indicated in this guidebook by Ⓐ, while nondesignated sites are indicated by ▲. The only section along the LSHT without a designated camping option is the 5.5-mile-long Section 11.

The LSHT often crosses or skirts private property. Use the trail descriptions, maps, and common sense when picking a camping spot. Disturbing or entering private property is illegal and only diminishes local support for the LSHT.

Campfires should be built only within existing fire rings; during dry seasons, campfires may be completely banned along the LSHT. Check with Sam Houston National Forest for any restrictions on open fires. (Backpacking stoves are typically, though not always, allowed during fire bans.) Anyone responsible for causing a wildfire is also responsible for all costs of fighting that fire; the USFS has been increasingly vigorous in prosecuting those linked to starting forest fires.

Hunting

Hunting is allowed throughout Sam Houston National Forest and on private property adjacent to and inside the forest. The only exception to this rule along the LSHT is that hunting is prohibited within **Big Creek and Winters Bayou Scenic Areas.**

Deer-hunting season varies each year but generally extends from late September to early January (the same dates when camping restrictions are in effect). Squirrel-hunting season is in March, and turkey-hunting season is typically in April. Hog-hunting season is year-round during daylight hours.

Hikers are advised to wear clothing in bright colors, such as fluorescent orange, during deer season. Hikers and hunters alike must camp in sites designated by the USFS during deer season.

Trail Ethics

We are only visitors in the wilderness. Preserving our wild lands requires that all who visit them use common sense and courtesy to ensure that no harm comes to them. Armed with a bit of knowledge and forethought, we can go into the woods, enjoy our trails and forests, and leave them pristine for those who follow. Before venturing out on the trail, refresh yourself on outdoor ethics.

Leave No Trace means that you must leave the woods in the same condition as (if not better condition than) before you arrived, with absolutely no trace of your passing. Small but harmful practices can accumulate over time so that what is only a trace of your passing today may become a destructive and ugly legacy as others follow your example in the future.

Stay on the trail even in muddy spots—walking around wet areas just widens the trail into an ugly mud pit. In some places the LSHT is routed adjacent to private property. Don't jump fences, camp in fields, or otherwise trespass on private land. Be courteous so that local landowners will continue to allow the trail to pass across their property.

Fires may be illegal and are extremely dangerous during dry seasons. Cook your backcountry meals using a backpacking stove. Campfires should be started only within existing fire rings. Don't cut live trees or branches; use only small downed pieces of wood. Always ensure that your campfire is completely extinguished when you're done cooking. If you must smoke, put out cigarettes and cigars completely (and pack out the butts with your trash).

Camp in previously used or established sites or in areas clear of vegetation and out of sight of the trail. If you must set up in a new and unused spot, pick a location at least 200 feet from the trail and at least 500 feet from water sources. If every hiker created a new tent site and fire ring, the trail would cease to feel like a backcountry experience.

Wildlife should be discouraged from visiting your camp and should not suffer any harm from your visit. Always keep a clean camp, and hang your food in trees away from easy access by raccoons. Leave wild animals alone, and never let your pets chase wildlife.

This rustic footbridge spans a creek near the trail's eastern terminus.

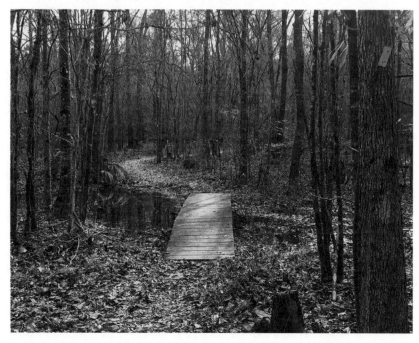

Human waste should be buried 4–6 inches deep, at least 100 feet from the trail, and at least 200 feet from creeks, rivers, or lakes. Pack out used toilet paper in zip-top plastic bags.

Litter is anything that you've brought with you into the woods—if you pack it in, you need to pack it out. Remember in particular that fruit peels, toilet paper, and cigarette butts take many years to degrade, and fire pits are not trash cans. It's a good practice to pick up any litter that you see, even if it's not yours.

Water is a precious resource and home to many fish and invertebrates. Don't put *anything* into any water source, even so-called biodegradable soap. Keep all bathroom activities far away from creeks, rivers, and lakes.

Dogs face more dangers and difficulties on the trail than humans. Ticks, chiggers, extreme heat, wildlife, and hunters all threaten a dog's health and safety. Keep dogs leashed and under your direct control on the trail and in camp. Provide plenty of water, and watch for signs of overexertion and heat stress.

Groups should be limited to six people or fewer. Larger groups not only greatly increase the possibility of damage to the trail, but they also decrease the solitude, the serenity, and the unique experience of being in the backcountry for both the group and other hikers they encounter.

Be quiet and considerate while you're hiking and in camp. Other people visit the backcountry to get away from the noise and bustle of city life. Don't use cell phones or other noise-generating technology near other people.

If you have any doubts, follow the hikers' golden rule: take only pictures, leave only footprints.

Thru-Hiking

Every year a few hikers set out to walk the entire length of the LSHT. Some hikers will piece together sections over time, perhaps even day-hiking the entire trail. *Thru-hikers* are generally defined as those who attempt a continuous, self-supported hike of the entire trail. Most thru-hikers will carry a loaded backpack and restock their food supplies somewhere along the way.

It's possible for an experienced, fit backpacker to thru-hike the LSHT without resupplying in as few as four or five days. Most thru-hikers, however, will walk at a pace that allows them to complete the trail in 8–10 days, and they will need to resupply about midway through their trek. Carrying enough food to thru-hike the entire trail is possible but not recommended—food is heavy, after all.

There are no resupply facilities directly along the LSHT, but **Huntsville State Park** and **Double Lake Recreation Area** both have small seasonal camp stores located within walking distance of the trail. A large gas station/convenience store is also a walkable distance from the trail in Section 11.

Hikers who are willing and able to travel by car from trail to town will find full-service grocery stores along the LSHT from Montgomery to Shepherd. Hikers can also mail themselves a package containing prepurchased resupply items, to be held in general delivery at the post office midway along the LSHT in Huntsville. Some hotels will also receive packages for guests who have room reservations, though this should be arranged well ahead of time. Each section description provides details on nearby resupply options, but thru-hikers will need to plan carefully in any case.

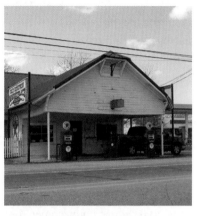

The town of New Waverly is 8 miles from the LSHT, but it offers hikers several options for dining and resupply.

Staging a food (or water) cache ahead of a thru-hike is also an option. Leave the cache out of sight of the trail but in a location you can easily remember and access. A hard plastic bucket with a lock-down or sealable lid should keep the weather and animals out of your food while it's hidden. Be sure to put your name and estimated date of pickup on the container, and always retrieve anything left after your hike.

Equipment

Selecting hiking equipment is a subjective process that depends on your personal experience and preferences. That said, there are some basic items that no hiker should be without when venturing into the woods. Appendix C (page 158) contains a checklist for day hikes and another for overnight trips. The lists are intended as a general guide; they include basic gear and some optional items but are not exhaustive.

If you're new to hiking, spend some time researching appropriate gear that will ensure safe and comfortable hiking in various seasons and trail conditions. Purchase (or rent) your gear from a reputable outdoors store that specializes in hiking and backpacking; don't try to cut corners by visiting a hunting and fishing store and purchasing heavy, often inadequate, equipment made for car camping. Good gear can make the difference between an enjoyable experience and a miserable—or even dangerous—ordeal.

Clothing

Always prepare for the worst: bring enough appropriate clothing to protect you from the most severe weather possible. Fast-moving cold fronts have been known to make temperatures in East Texas dip more than 40° within a few hours. Add in heavy rains and high winds, and you have a recipe for hypothermia, a potentially dangerous drop in body temperature. Note that it doesn't take freezing temperatures for hypothermia to set in.

"Cotton kills" is a common saying among hikers in cold climates, but it's just as applicable in East Texas: walking in wet cotton clothes on a 45° day can easily bring on hypothermia. The key to enjoyable hiking on the LSHT is to layer synthetic clothing. A synthetic shirt, sweater, or fleece jacket, plus an outer shell, will keep you both warmer and drier than a single heavy outer layer. Shedding or adding layers helps your body regulate its temperature more effectively than a single heavy jacket. Synthetic fabrics dry quickly and maintain their insulating properties when wet; even in the heat of the summer, it's advisable to wear lightweight synthetic clothing that will dry in the humid conditions of the LSHT. Lightweight long pants and a long-sleeve shirt will protect you from the sun, biting insects, and thorny brush that can overhang the trail.

Footwear

Many a hiking trip has been ruined because of blisters. Footwear is a personal choice that may take some experimenting to master. I prefer to wear midweight leather hiking boots, as well as knee-high synthetic gaiters to keep mud off my pants, keep dirt out of my boots, and protect my lower legs from sharp brush and snakes. Many hikers prefer low-top trail hikers that resemble running shoes; low-cut gaiters are also available. Whatever your choice of footwear, remember to break in your shoes before you get on the trail. And don't neglect to purchase high-quality socks made expressly for hiking—on a multiday outing, carry two or three pairs of wool–synthetic blend socks. Finally, consider purchasing high-quality insoles for maximum support.

Sleeping Bags and Pads

A bag rated to 30°F or 40°F will probably be enough for most hikers in the fall and spring. I prefer to carry a warmer sleeping bag (one rated to 20°F) most of the year because I sleep cold. Midsummer on the LSHT can bring extremely hot daytime temperatures, but most people will need at least a light fleece blanket for camping even in July and August. Summer sleeping bags are lightweight and low cost. Don't forget to bring a sleeping pad, which makes all the difference in warmth and comfort. Pads come in many styles and materials, from cheaper closed-cell foam to the more costly inflatable versions. I've used them all and haven't noticed a big difference in comfort among the varieties available.

Tents and Hammocks

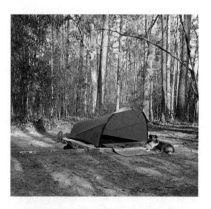

Because of the prolific insect population in East Texas, I advise using an enclosed tent versus the more open design of a tarp. I've used tarps extensively—I've even slept out in the open under the stars—in dry desert climates, with good results. I tried using a tarp on the LSHT in January, and even though I didn't see any insects during the day and experienced cold temperatures at night, I had to share my sleeping space with a parade of spiders and ants. In warmer seasons,

This lightweight backpacking tent is the author's home on the trail.

mosquitoes and ticks make an enclosed tent a necessity for comfort.

Hammocks make an excellent sleeping choice on the LSHT. Well-spaced trees are easy to find, though occasionally the underbrush may prove too tall or thick to make putting up a hammock practical. Ensuring that your hammock has adequate rain and bug protection is essential for comfort, just as with tents. Hikers who prefer hammock camping will find that the LSHT offers nearly limitless options—so many, in fact, that I didn't have room to list them all in this guidebook. Know, however, that most of the tent-camping sites listed here are good potential hammock-camping spots as well, because they have little or no ground cover.

Water Treatment

All water sources harbor microorganisms capable of making you very ill, so carry water-purification tablets made of iodine or a chlorine compound (the cheapest option) and/or a filter made specifically for hikers. Portable ultraviolet-light purifiers work only with clear water, so be sure to use a pre-filter of some kind in conjunction with them. With proper treatment, just about any water along the LSHT is safe to drink; unless you find yourself in an emergency, however, you'll want to avoid filtering or treating very stagnant water or runoff that may be contaminated by chemicals or livestock waste.

Food

Novice hikers often make the mistake of carrying too much food. If you aren't accustomed to the exertion of backpacking, your appetite may actually decrease

Cotton Creek Cemetery Road leads hikers past pleasant open fields at the end of the Conroe Section. Photo: James Weatherby

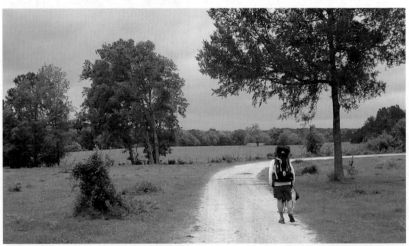

for the first day or two. On the other hand, it's a good idea to carry a day of extra food in case you get stranded by bad weather or other trouble; 2 pounds of food per person, per day, is the average. Many lightweight backpacking staples can be purchased at a grocery store; you need not rely on expensive prepared backpacking food sold at outdoors stores. See Appendix C (page 158) for specific backpacking food ideas.

Hazards and Personal Safety

Like many outdoor activities, hiking inherently involves some risk. The following is a brief rundown of the most common safety concerns for LSHT hikers. For more-detailed information, check out classes and books dedicated to wilderness first aid.

Heat

Heat exhaustion and heatstroke are potentially deadly threats on the LSHT in summer. Carry plenty of water at all times. Take frequent rest breaks when high humidity combines with heat to make it hard to stay cool. Consider hiking only in the lower temperatures of early morning and late evening.

Insects

While bugs are more of an inconvenience than a threat, LSHT hikers are more likely to have an uncomfortable encounter with these creatures than with any other. Both ticks and mosquitoes can carry potentially life-threatening diseases and are present during every month of the year in the moist forests of East Texas.

During April–September, the worst months for bugs, carry insect repellent and consider wearing long pants. After the first freezing night of the year, usually sometime in October, ticks and mosquitoes mostly disappear until the next spring—again, though, they never go away completely.

It's a good idea to check for ticks each evening. Removing ticks before they have a chance to feed is crucial, as several diseases are transmitted only after the tick has been attached at least 24 hours. The diseases that can be transmitted to humans by infected ticks in Texas are Lyme disease, Rocky Mountain spotted fever, ehrlichiosis, and relapsing fever. If caught early, these diseases can be successfully treated, but if left untreated they can be serious or even fatal.

Early symptoms may include a rash around the bite or flulike symptoms, such as fever, headache, fatigue, muscle aches, and joint pain.

Chiggers are tiny mites, nearly invisible to humans, which can cause a lot of torment. Most numerous in the spring, chiggers bite into the skin (often around the folds of the body, like the knees or waistline) and cause hard, red welts that itch intensely for up to a week. Your best bet to avoid chiggers is to not sit directly on the ground in the spring and early summer, especially in sunny, grassy areas. Use your tent's ground cloth—or bring along a piece of light plastic—to spread on the ground before you sit down for a break.

Two venomous spider species are found in East Texas: the black widow and the brown recluse. Both species are solitary and live in sheltered areas such as underneath logs or in thick bushes. Be particularly cautious when you leave the trail to relieve yourself or collect firewood—watch where you put your hands. The spiders that build their webs directly across the trail can bite but are not venomous.

Other bothersome insects that hikers may encounter on the LSHT are flies and gnats, especially in mid-to-late summer. Fire ants are also present but typically live in open areas—watch for their telltale mounds in power-line rights-of-way and fields, especially during or after rain when water over the trail may cause fire ants to swarm. Of course, bees and wasps are active in all of the warmer months and a serious concern for anyone allergic to their stings.

Snakes

For some hikers, snakes are a major worry. The fact is, though, that snakes pose no real threat to humans—lightning strikes, drowning, and hunting accidents are much more common outdoor hazards. Snakes are an extremely important part of a healthy ecosystem, keeping the population of rodents and small animals in balance. Of the more than 30 species of snakes in East Texas, only a few are venomous: the water moccasin, rattlesnake, copperhead, and coral snake. Look before you sit on logs or against the base of trees. Never reach blindly under logs or into brush. Most snake bites occur on the hands or feet.

Spotting a snake in its natural environment should be treated just like any other wildlife encounter. Keep your distance. Don't kill or try to capture snakes—it's harmful to the environment and potentially harmful to you! Another consideration: federal and state laws protect a few species of East Texas snakes that are listed as threatened, subjecting violators to fines up to $100,000 or one year of imprisonment.

If the worst happens and you think you've been bitten by a venomous snake, it's important to reach help with a minimum of exertion. Use your maps to find the nearest exit to civilization. Walk out calmly—don't run. Avoid moving the bitten limb more than necessary, and remove any rings or constrictive jewelry before swelling begins. On average, fewer than 1% of all snakebites recorded in the US are fatal.

Animals

In East Texas, bears, jaguars, cougars, and wolves were hunted to extinction by 1950. Coyotes and bobcats are the most numerous large predators in the East Texas woods today; both are extremely timid and will not bother humans. Raccoons are the animal that is probably most likely to invade hikers' camps in their nightly hunt for food. Store food in animal-proof canisters, or in trees away from trunks, to keep it out of reach.

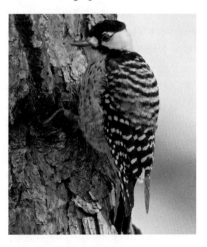

Most mammals, from coyotes and foxes to skunks and bats, can carry rabies. Do not approach or handle *any* wild animals—for their safety and yours.

The American alligator has returned in healthy numbers to its home range on the waterways of East Texas. Although they appear frightening, alligators are known to be shy around humans. LSHT hikers have little to fear from them. The best places to watch for

The LSHT passes through some of the last habitat left for the endangered red-cockaded woodpecker (*Picoides borealis*).

Photo: feathercollector/Shutterstock

the seldom-seen alligators are around the shoreline of Lake Conroe, near Stubblefield Lake, and in the larger waterways, like the San Jacinto River.

Humans

It's a statistical fact that the most dangerous animal encounter a hiker can have is with another human. Hunting accidents happen every year. Even though it's illegal to discharge a weapon across or down a trail corridor, road, or campground, you can't rule out the possibility that a hunter may fire in your direction or mistake you for an animal. Wear brightly colored clothing during rifle-hunting deer season (November–January) to increase your visibility to hunters.

Keep a low profile when hiking. Don't make yourself an easy target for harassment, even though the odds of a person bothering you on the LSHT are extremely low. It's always a good practice not to camp near roads—unless you are in a developed campground—and to camp out of sight of the trail. The idea is not to be paranoid but to be smart. Watch for traffic while crossing or walking on roads.

Plants

Keep an eye out for poison ivy and poison oak; both are prolific along the LSHT and cause contact dermatitis in most people. Poison ivy is a climbing vine of three leaflets that grows almost straight up instead of twining around its support. Eastern poison oak does indeed have multilobed leaves that resemble oak and can be found in moist, sandy soils. Poison sumac, although not common along the LSHT, is a water-loving tree commonly found in swamps; it grows between 6 and 20 feet tall, with compound leaves that turn bright red and yellow in the fall. Consult photos of each of these plants before you venture into the East Texas woodland so you can identify them. The branches of these plants (usually bare in winter) can also be poisonous.

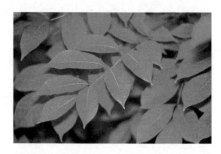

Poison sumac
Photo: Norman Tomalin/Alamy Stock Photo

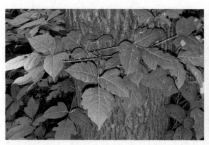

Poison ivy
Photo: Tom Watson

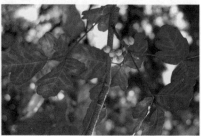

Poison oak
Photo: Jane Huber

Prescribed Burns

The USFS sets fire to tracts, or compartments, of the Sam Houston National Forest on a rotating basis depending on how much underbrush and fallen limbs have built up, along with wind direction and weather conditions. Look for advance notice of prescribed burns on the Sam Houston National Forest and LSHTC websites.

Prescribed burns are rarely fast-moving, intense, or dangerous, but they do generate a lot of smoke that can irritate eyes and lungs. Burns are often conducted in late winter or early spring. In addition to announce burns online, the USFS will also post signs along the LSHT closing the trail for 24 hours where a burn crosses the trail. Stumps will often smolder and ash can cover ponds and slow-moving creeks for days.

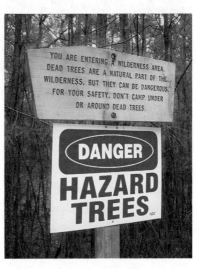

Falling Trees and Limbs

The LSHT's woods are so thick that a hiker may find nowhere to escape falling limbs and trees during high winds. Pine trees have particularly soft wood that splinters easily. Some areas along the trail may even have warnings posted at trailheads informing hikers where there are many standing dead or diseased trees. Always check overhead before pitching a tent in the woods.

A warning sign posted in LSHT Section 1, Wilderness

Watch out for dead limbs or trees (aka "widowmakers") that could fall during the night. Don't venture into the woods during windstorms or when high winds are forecast. If you find yourself in the woods during windy conditions, take refuge in a gully or beside large fallen tree trunks that can offer some protection.

Rising Creeks

Heavy rains can cause large creeks and rivers to rise rapidly out of their banks. Dry creek beds and drainages that were once dry may fill up. Bottomlands can

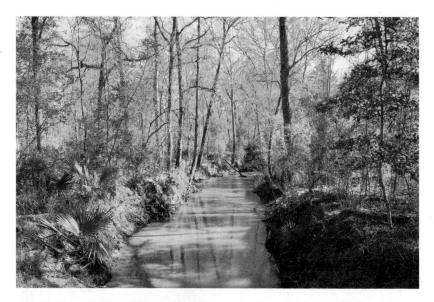

Caney Creek (see Section 2, page 51) may be dry after a long summer.

turn into extensive swamps. If you have any doubts about crossing high water, either turn around or be patient and stay put on dry ground until the water recedes (it may take more than a day or two). During extended periods of rain in late winter, it may be necessary to detour around flooded areas. However, many sections of the LSHT are located on higher, upland areas away from bottomlands and can be hiked even in very wet weather. Consult the section information in Chapter 3 to identify potential problem areas.

Getting Lost . . . or Misplaced

If you've been walking along the trail and you haven't seen any trail markers after about 5 minutes of hiking, you may want to turn around and retrace your steps until you find a marker—you may have missed a turn in the trail. It's possible that a few trail markers are missing in a section due to vandalism or fallen trees, but the LSHT hiker should never walk more than 5 minutes without seeing a marker. (A hiker can estimate covering 1 mile in about 30 minutes.) Most of the LSHT road walks are not regularly marked, though, so don't expect to see LSHT trail markers while on roads. Instead, watch your maps and use this book to find your way on road walks.

The forests along the LSHT are often thick and sometimes look the same in every direction, so it is imperative not to wander off the trail into the woods where it's easy to become disoriented. In the event that you do become lost, you have several important decisions to make and some basic guidelines to follow.

First, keep calm. Consider yourself misplaced for a bit, not lost. Take a break to think about how long you've been misplaced, what direction you've come from, and what information your map may be able to provide about your location. Very few places along the LSHT are more than a couple of miles of walking from a road, utilities right-of-way, or some form of civilization. Keep your backpack and gear with you at all times. If you're on a trail, don't leave it—it will lead you somewhere much faster and with less danger than trying to walk into the woods off-trail. If you're injured, it's getting dark, or you're panicked or exhausted, make camp and stay put, at least for the night. As a last resort, if you do become lost in deep woods off-trail, follow drainages downstream, or follow utilities or pipeline right-of-ways—eventually, they'll lead you to a trail or road.

It's in every hiker's best interest to read a few resources that explain what to do in case you get misplaced while hiking. Always carry maps and a compass, and tell someone back in civilization where you're hiking and when you expect to return home.

Cell Phone Coverage

The remote nature and uninterrupted tree canopy of Sam Houston National Forest mean that cellular coverage is extremely limited along most of the trail, so don't rely on your phone for location or calling services while hiking the LSHT.

Before You Go

In summary, before you set out on an LSHT hike of any distance, check news reports and also check with the LSHTC and Sam Houston National Forest for the following: (1) weather conditions, including drought status or, conversely, recent rainfall activity in the region; (2) trail closures, including any major bridges that may be out; (3) hunting-season restrictions, if applicable; (4) news and announcements regarding USFS prescribed burns; and (5) water levels at the crossing of the East Fork of the San Jacinto River if the hiker bridge is still out in Section 8. Plan for insect activity and, most importantly, dress and pack for worst-case weather.

CHAPTER THREE

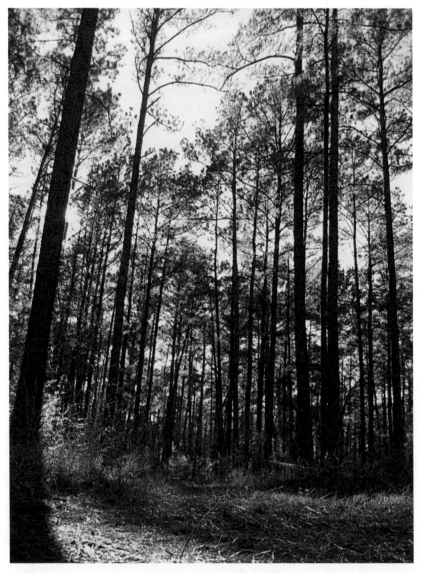

Tall pines line the Wilderness Section of the LSHT.

TRAIL
SECTIONS

||||||||||||||||||||||||||||||||||||||||||||||||||||||||||||||||||||||||||||||||||||||||||||||||||||||||||||||||||||||||||||

SECTION 1: WILDERNESS 8.7 MILES

**FARM TO MARKET 149 NEAR RICHARDS
TO FARM TO MARKET 149 CROSSING**

OVERVIEW

THE WILDERNESS SECTION of the Lone Star Hiking Trail
(LSHT) is so named because it passes through the only officially designated wilderness area on the trail: 3,855-acre
Little Lake Creek Wilderness, established in 1984. Protected
hardwood bottomland drainages, like Little Lake Creek, are
becoming rare because of pressure from development, agriculture, logging, and reservoir-building. Little Lake Creek
and its seasonally flowing tributaries harbor fertile soils,
wetlands, and unique tree species: an important sanctuary
for resident wildlife and migrating waterfowl.

Hikers in the Wilderness Section experience upland
pine forests, meandering creeks, palmetto flats, and seasonal
swamps. Water is plentiful, but extensive boardwalks keep
feet dry in most wet areas. Section 1 is both well maintained
and easily accessible. A variety of hiking trails in the area
can be linked to make loop hikes along the LSHT; hikers
must pay close attention to maps and trail markers to avoid
winding up on the wrong path.

A detailed *Little Lake Creek Wilderness* map can be
ordered from the U.S. Forest Service; a map and concise
trail guide are also available at the website for the Lone Star
Hiking Trail Club (LSHTC), lonestartrail.org.

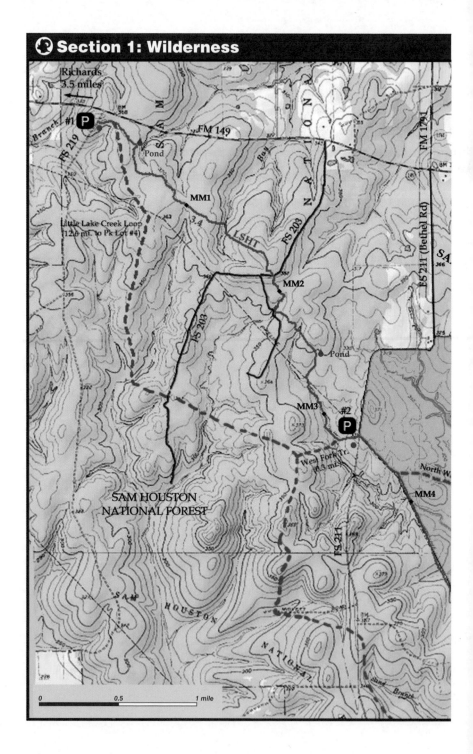

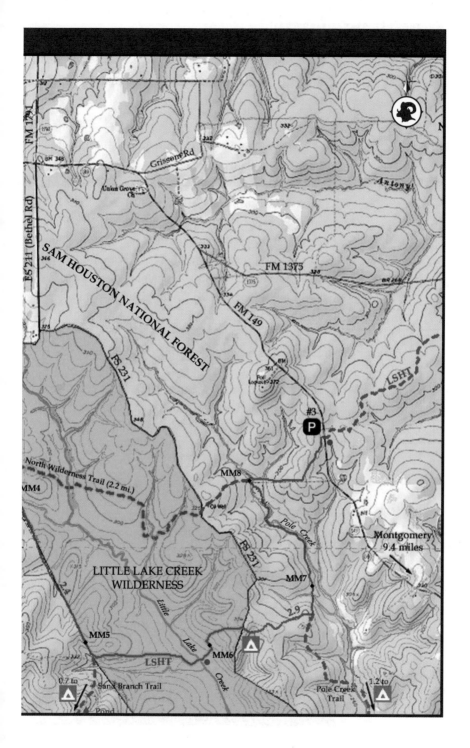

TRAIL ACCESS AND PARKING

Section 1 offers hikers three trailheads with plenty of room for parking; each is located on, or accessed from, Farm to Market (FM) 149, designated on signs as Farm Road 149. Drinking water is unavailable at the trailheads.

The western terminus of the LSHT is **Richards Trailhead Parking Lot 1,** about 3 miles east of the small town of Richards and 14.5 miles north of Montgomery. Look for dirt Forest Service (FS) Road 219 on the south side of FM 149. Trailhead Parking Lot 1 is on the left, just 0.1 mile down FS 219. A brown sign on the highway indicates the turnoff for the LSHT, but the parking lot isn't visible from FM 149.

Trailhead Parking Lot 2, also called **Sandy Branch,** offers access at trail mile 3.4. Roughly midway between Trailhead Parking Lots 1 and 3 along FM 149, about 12 miles north of Montgomery, turn onto FS 211/ Bethel Road, on the south side of FM 149; *note:* there

A small store in Richards provides hikers with a place to grab last-minute supplies and lunch.

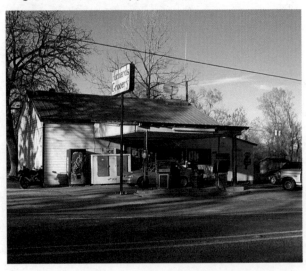

is no sign for the LSHT at this turn. Trailhead Parking Lot 2 is located on the west side of FS 211, approximately 2 miles from FM 149.

A third trailhead, **North Wilderness Trailhead Parking Lot 3,** is located on FM 149 about 9.5 miles north of Montgomery, where the LSHT crosses FM 149 at trail mile 8.7 at the end of LSHT Section 1. This parking area is signed and visible from the highway.

A potential source of confusion is a fourth trailhead that is signed LONE STAR HIKING TRAIL but actually connects to the LSHT via the Little Lake Creek Loop Trail. This fourth trailhead, **Parking Lot 4,** 6.9 miles north of Montgomery, is the first one you'll see as you drive north on FM 149 from Montgomery.

SECTION 1 GPS Waypoints	
LSHT Richards Trailhead Parking Lot 1, FM 149	N30° 32.317' W95° 47.090'
LSHT Sandy Branch Trailhead Parking Lot 2, FS 211	N30° 30.637' W95° 45.420'
Crossing of Little Lake Creek at LSHT mile 5.9	N30° 29.405' W95° 43.851'
LSHT North Wilderness Trailhead Parking Lot 3, FM 149	N30° 30.610' W95° 43.079'
Trailhead Parking Lot at Little Lake Creek Loop Trail, FM 149 (not main LSHT)	N30° 28.912' W95° 41.840'

SUPPLIES AND ACCOMMODATIONS

Richards (population 296) is 3 miles west of LSHT Trailhead Parking Lot 1 (the trail's western terminus) on FM 149. The town's amenities are limited to two bar-and-grill taverns (open only on weekends and located along FM 149 just 2 miles from Parking Lot 1), a post office, and a small grocery store with deli (lunch served 11 a.m.–1:30 p.m., seven days a week).

Historic **Montgomery** (population 621) is located 9.4 miles south of LSHT Trailhead Parking Lot 3, at trail mile 8.7 at the eastern end of Section 1—at the junction of FM 149 and Texas State Highway (TX) 105. This rapidly growing town offers more hiker-resupply options than Richards, including a full-size grocery store, several restaurants and fast-food places, gas stations, and many other businesses. At least one bed-and-breakfast offers overnight lodging in Montgomery.

Finally, **Conroe** (population: 82,286), 15 miles east of Montgomery on TX 105 along I-45, offers a wide range of overnight lodging and services.

WATER

The westernmost half of Section 1 harbors two small forest ponds, one of which is drought-resistant. The trail crosses a small spring-fed creek near mile 4 that flows year-round, unlike seasonal Little Lake Creek and its wetlands near mile 6. You can expect to find water in this section even during extreme droughts.

TRAIL DESCRIPTION

The LSHT begins in Sam Houston National Forest beneath a canopy of tall loblolly pines interspersed with the occasional oak or hickory. Soon after leaving the western terminus, you reach a well-signed intersection, with the orange-blazed Little Lake Creek Loop heading off to the right. This trail, often called The Grand Loop, is known for its many ponds, creeks, and wetland areas, making it a beautiful trek; its eastern end is sometimes too boggy to walk in wet seasons, however. Little Lake Creek passes Parking Lot 4 in 12.6 miles and eventually ends in 18.5 miles at an intersection with the LSHT in Section 2.

At 0.3 mile the LSHT jogs to the left at a utilities right-of-way, passing a short side trail to a small but

picturesque pond, ◊◊◊ visible in the pines to the left of   ◊ **Water**
the trail and sporting its own bird-watching bench. For a
few hundred feet on either side of **MILE MARKER 1** (elevation 363'), open areas in a mature forest of oaks and pines,
interspersed with rough jeep tracks, offer possible waterless camping. ▲ As you pass these open sites, the forest   ▲ **Campsite**
undergrowth becomes thicker, limiting camping opportunities until the first creek drainage.

You'll enter pure stands of immature pines interspersed with what appear to be old clear-cuts. In April 2015
high winds in this area toppled 128 large trees, which were
later salvaged and sold by the U.S. Forest Service.

Cross gravel FS 203 and a small seasonal stream just
before **MILE MARKER 2**; then follow the creek in a wilder,
more scenic forest. Be careful at mile 2.1 to follow the blazes
to the left—and remember that if you're hiking westbound,
you need to reverse all directions, left and right, in these
trail descriptions—heading east-southeast, paralleling dirt
FS 203 but not crossing it; note that there may be some con-
flicting blazes leading northward to the road.

Pass over a rough logging road and through an open,
grassy area beneath smaller trees. Then top out on a rise
under towering pines, and pass a small pond ◊◊◊◊◊ at   ◊ **Water**
mile 2.5 with overgrown banks that offers minimal space
for camping. ▲   ▲ **Campsite**

After the pond, the trail parallels a couple of creek
drainages and then passes some bull pines. The drainage
becomes deeper and more apt to hold water as you follow
it past **MILE MARKER 3**. There is some relief to the land in
the form of several small rises.

At a crossing of the drainage, you'll reach the junction with the West Fork Trail, which turns off to the right
and is marked with blue-and-purple-striped blazes. At
mile 3.4, cross gravel road FS 211, where LSHT Trailhead Parking Lot 2 is visible to the right. Sign the hiker

register at the road before entering Little Lake Creek Wilderness. Watch for Eastern red cedar adjacent to the trail just inside the Wilderness. At mile 3.5, past a dense stand of baby pines, a clearing off to the right offers potential **Campsite ▲** camping **▲** out of sight of the road. A boardwalk leads over a wetland, but just a short distance later a section of unbridged trail near mile 3.7 can be muddy. Signs at mile 3.8 mark the junction of the red-blazed, 2.2-mile North Wilderness Trail, which heads off to the left and intersects the LSHT again at Mile Marker 8.

Just before **MILE MARKER 4**, pass a clear, spring-fed **Water ◊** creek ◊◊◊◊ and another solitary Eastern red cedar tree. Ignore a small section of LSHT that splits into two paths—either way leads quickly to the same outcome. Smooth alder, also called black alder, grows along these bottomlands; in fall and winter, look for its bare branches tipped with tiny "cones." A relatively small deciduous tree growing to 40 feet in height, black alder often grows in thickets at the edge of wetlands and is one of the few tree species that can fix atmospheric nitrogen through bacteria in its roots.

At mile 4.5 cross a creek that flows with clear water in the cooler seasons. At mile 4.7, an open area to the right amid well-spaced pines could make an acceptable **Campsite ▲** dry camp. **▲** Gradually, you leave the hardwoods, cross open bottomland where you spot your first dwarf palmettos (*Sabal minor*), and then climb into a pleasant upland among giant pines. The rolling landscape drops again into swampy palmetto bottomlands just before **MILE MARKER 5**. Reach a signed junction with the yellow-blazed Sand Branch Trail, which heads straight ahead while the LSHT makes a left turn. By following the Sand Branch Trail for 0.7 mile, you can reach a designated (approved for use during deer-hunting season) primitive backpacker campsite, Sand Branch Camp, and a picturesque open area around **Campsite Ⓐ** Sand Branch Pond. Ⓐ

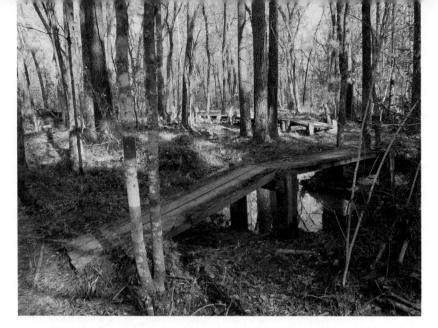

Boy Scout–constructed boardwalks span Little Lake Creek.

Over the next mile, you'll be happy to walk on a series of boardwalks built by Boy Scouts. The scenic bottomlands surrounding Little Lake Creek ⬥ can become a large swamp at times, hiding the creek's exact whereabouts somewhere just before **MILE MARKER 6**. Yaupon, alder, and other wetland-loving vegetation flourish here, along with a diverse bird population. At mile 6.4, a sign lets you know that you're leaving Little Lake Creek Wilderness and also points the way (left) down unsigned FS 231, 0.2 mile to a small designated backpacker campsite with no water source but room for several tents. ⬥ Heading out of the wilderness boundaries, the young forest has a few huge pine trees with large duff mounds around their bases.

⬥ Water

⬥ Campsite

The LSHT makes a sharp left turn at mile 6.7—this is the junction with the blue-blazed Pole Creek Trail, a mile down which is a designated backpacker campsite and a meeting with the Little Lake Creek Loop. ⬥ Parking Lot 4 can be reached 2.3 miles from this junction with the LSHT by first following the Pole Creek Trail and then turning left and heading east for another mile down the Little Lake Creek Loop.

⬥ Campsite

As you near **MILE MARKER 7**, pass a farm and begin walking downhill along an old barbwire-fence line. Around the private property, expect to hear dogs barking—don't plan to camp in the vicinity. You quickly return to a peaceful hardwood forest broken by numerous creeks, one of which the trail follows. There are a few places to scramble **Water** down the banks to access water at mile 7.2. Potential **Campsite** campsites border the creek, although undergrowth becomes thicker at mile 7.5. Here, native dwarf palmettos, the first magnolias seen along the trail, and hanging vines lend a junglelike feel to the woods. Just past the bridge at **MILE MARKER 8**, turn right to stay on the LSHT at the junction with the red-blazed North Wilderness Trail, which heads to the left back to its junction with the LSHT at mile 3.8. Immediately, you encounter sandy-bottomed Pole Creek; crossing it usually entails a large hop over a **Water** few inches of clear water, though it can be a difficult ford after heavy rain. As you gradually climb out of the creek bottom, look for river birch and white oaks before returning to mature upland pine forest. You may hear traffic on FM 149 for nearly a mile before you reach the trailhead and LSHT Trailhead Parking Lot 3 at mile 8.7. Section 2 of the LSHT continues across the highway.

Many trees were damaged or toppled after high winds hit the western end of Section 1 in 2015.

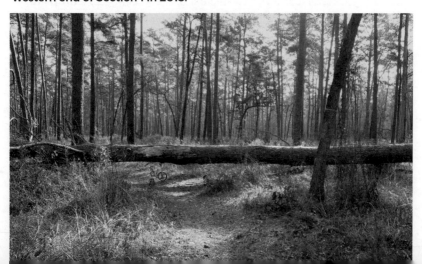

SECTION 1 Mileage

MILES W→E	TRAIL POINT	MILES E→W	NOTES
0.0	Western terminus of LSHT, FS 219 at FM 149, LSHT Richards Trailhead Parking Lot 1	96.4	▭ P
0.1	Little Lake Creek Loop Trail (orange-blazed) branches right; left on LSHT	96.3	
0.2	Utilities right-of-way	96.2	
0.3	Small pond (semiclear water ◊◊◊)	96.1	◊
0.4	Seasonal drainage on left	96.0	
1.0	**MILE MARKER 1**; potential camping	95.4	▲
1.3	Large seasonal drainage	95.1	
1.8	FS 203 (good dirt road)	94.6	▭
2.0	Small seasonal drainage; **MILE MARKER 2**	94.4	
2.1	Left on LSHT, parallel to FS 203	94.3	▭
2.2	Abandoned jeep road	94.2	
2.5	Small pond (semiclear water ◊◊◊◊◊); potential camping	93.9	◊ ▲
2.7	Large seasonal drainage	93.7	
3.0	**MILE MARKER 3**	93.4	
3.3	Junction with West Fork Trail (purple-blazed); large seasonal drainage	93.1	
3.4	FS 211 (good gravel road); LSHT Sandy Branch Trailhead Parking Lot 2; enter Little Lake Creek (LLC) Wilderness	93.0	▭ P
3.5	Potential camping	92.9	▲
3.8	Wilderness Trail branches left (red-blazed); straight on LSHT	92.6	
4.0	**MILE MARKER 4;** creek (low volume, good water ◊◊◊◊)	92.4	◊
4.5	Large seasonal drainage (stagnant water)	91.9	
4.7	Potential camping	91.7	▲
5.0	**MILE MARKER 5**	91.4	
5.1	Intersect Sand Branch Trail (yellow-blazed; 0.5 mi+ to primitive camping and pond); left on LSHT	91.3	Ⓐ
5.9	Boardwalks over Little Lake Creek bottomland ◊	90.5	◊

continued on next page

SECTION 1 Mileage

MILES W→E	TRAIL POINT	MILES E→W	NOTES
6.0	**MILE MARKER 6**	90.4	
6.4	LLC Wilderness boundary; FS 231 (0.2 mi to designated camping)	90.0	▬ Ⓐ
6.7	Pole Creek Trail (blue-blazed) heads right; left on LSHT	89.7	
7.0	**MILE MARKER 7**	89.4	
7.2	Creek adjacent to trail (low volume, good water ⚊)	89.2	🚰
7.7	Hiker bridge over deep drainage	88.7	
8.0	**MILE MARKER 8;** Pole Creek (low volume, good water); junction with North Wilderness Trail	88.4	▬ 🚰
8.6	Utilities right-of-way	87.8	
8.7	FM 149, LSHT North Wilderness Trailhead Parking Lot 3	87.7	▬ 🅿

MILEAGE CHART KEY

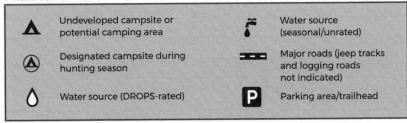

🔺 Undeveloped campsite or potential camping area

Ⓐ Designated campsite during hunting season

💧 Water source (DROPS-rated)

🚰 Water source (seasonal/unrated)

▬▬▬ Major roads (jeep tracks and logging roads not indicated)

🅿 Parking area/trailhead

Shaded by mature pine trees, numerous open areas are conducive to tents and hammocks in Section 1 during seasons when backcountry camping is allowed.

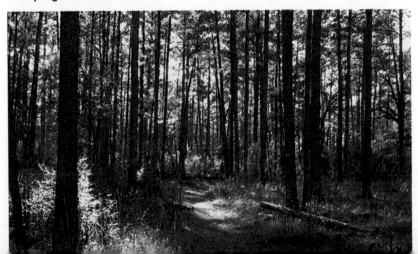

**FARM TO MARKET 149 CROSSING
TO FARM TO MARKET 1375**

OVERVIEW

HIKERS IN THE KELLY SECTION will enjoy walking through a wide variety of forest communities. The Caney Creek bottomlands in particular offer an enjoyable mix of tree species and plant communities that harbor an abundance of birds and wildlife.

This section has few reliable water sources for overnight hikers but tends to remain muddy in many areas. All large creeks are bridged, and the trail continues to be easy to follow, with abundant trail markers and signs. There are plenty of high and dry campsites to be found along the way, though hikers may need to carry water to camp.

The intersection of the Lone Star Hiking Trail (LSHT) and the Little Lake Creek Loop Trail offers hikers a chance to walk an 18.5-mile loop that connects the LSHT in Sections 1 and 2. A detailed *Little Lake Creek Wilderness* map can be ordered from the U.S. Forest Service (USFS); a map and concise trail guide are also available at lonestartrail.org.

TRAIL ACCESS AND PARKING

Section 2 offers hikers two official LSHT trailhead parking areas. The western end of Section 2, at mile 8.7, has parking in **LSHT North Wilderness Trailhead Parking Lot 3,** on Farm to Market (FM) 149 (designated on signs as Farm Road 149), about 9.5 miles north of Montgomery where the LSHT crosses FM 149.

The eastern end of Section 2 offers hiker parking at **LSHT Stubblefield Trailhead Parking Lot 6,** just off FM 1375 down a small dirt access road (the parking lot isn't visible from the highway) at LSHT mile 15.8. Both parking areas/trail crossings are well signed. Additionally, several cars could park trailside at the LSHT crossing of Osborn Road/Forest Service Road (FS) 237 at mile 11.3 and at the trail crossing of FS 271 (just off FS 204) at mile 14.2. Water is unavailable at the trailheads.

SECTION 2 GPS Waypoints	
LSHT North Wilderness Trailhead Parking Lot 3, FM 149	N30° 30.610' W95° 43.079'
LSHT Caney Creek Trailhead Parking Lot 4, Little Lake Creek Loop	N30° 28.912' W95° 41.840'
LSHT Crossing of Osborn Rd., mile 11.3	N30° 31.221' W95° 41.064'
Crossing of Caney Creek, mile 11.9	N30° 31.241' W95° 40.619'
LSHT Crossing of FS 271/FS 204, mile 14.2	N30° 31.172' W95° 40.849'
LSHT Stubblefield Trailhead Parking Lot 6, FM 1375	N30° 31.563' W95 °37.812'

SUPPLIES AND ACCOMMODATIONS

Montgomery (population 621) is 9.4 miles south of North Wilderness Trailhead Parking Lot 3 on FM 149 at the beginning of Section 2. The town has a full-size grocery store, several restaurants, gas stations, and many other businesses. At least one bed-and-breakfast offers overnight lodging in Montgomery.

Conroe (population 82,286), 15 miles east of Montgomery on Texas State Highway (TX) 105 along I-45, offers a wide variety of overnight lodging and services.

At the end of Section 2, **New Waverly** (population 1,032) lies about 9 miles east of Stubblefield Parking Lot 6 on FM 1375, just east of I-45. New Waverly has no overnight lodging but does host several combination gas stations/convenience stores, restaurants, an auto-parts store, a library, and a grocery store. From New Waverly, it's 15 miles north on I-45 to the full-service town of **Huntsville,** which offers many options for overnight lodging.

WATER

Water is not as regular in Section 2 as it is in Section 1. Plan your hike carefully if you need water for camping. Although there are plenty of campsites, most of them are in dry areas. The most reliable water source in this section is a pond just off the trail that is difficult for hikers to spot, at mile 9.8. The Caney Creek crossing at mile 11.9 will be dry at the end of long summers or during prolonged droughts.

TRAIL DESCRIPTION

Section 2 begins at LSHT Trailhead Parking Lot 3, on FM 149 at mile 8.7. From this dirt lot, as you stand near the information board, look directly across FM 149—you should be able to see the trail marked on the other side of the highway where it heads into the woods.

After crossing FM 149, the trail swings left along an old barbwire fence, crosses a jeep track, and makes a hard right turn. (Remember that if you're hiking westbound, you need to reverse all directions, left and right, in these trail descriptions.) At mile 8.9 you reach a junction of trails where the blazes may be hard for eastbound trekkers to see—the LSHT makes a sharp left turn here. Shortly after the turn, **MILE MARKER 9** is visible on a tree to the right of the trail. Again, at mile 9.1, the LSHT makes another hard turn—this one to the left—as it reaches a faint jeep track that continues straight. It would be easy to miss this turn, so watch carefully.

Yet another junction of trails at mile 9.3 is clearly marked; the LSHT heads left and soon reaches some flat land in an open forest that could be used for waterless camping. ▲ At mile 9.6 the trail begins to skirt a pine forest to the right but stays within the canopy of the larger oak–pine forest to the left. If it has been raining a lot, there

▲ Campsite

53

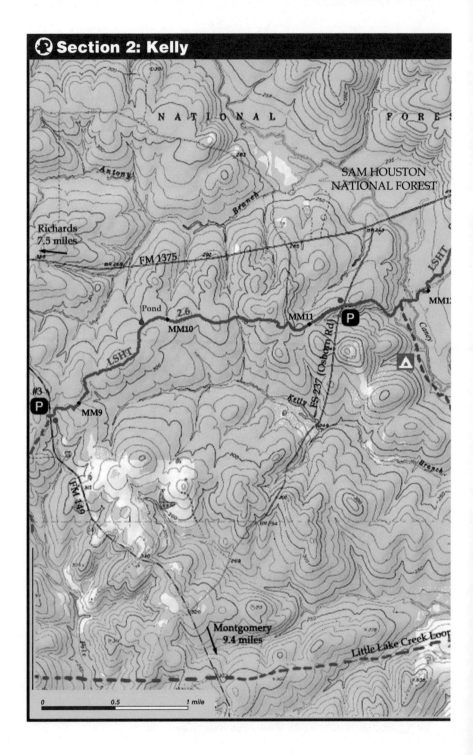

SAM HOUSTON
NATIONAL FOREST

Richards
7.5 miles

FM 1375

Pond   2.6

MM10

MM11

P

MM1...

LSHT

Caney

#3

P

MM9

Kelly

FS 237 (Osburn Rd)

Branch

FM 149

Mt.

Montgomery
9.4 miles

Little Lake Creek Loop

0   0.5   1 mile

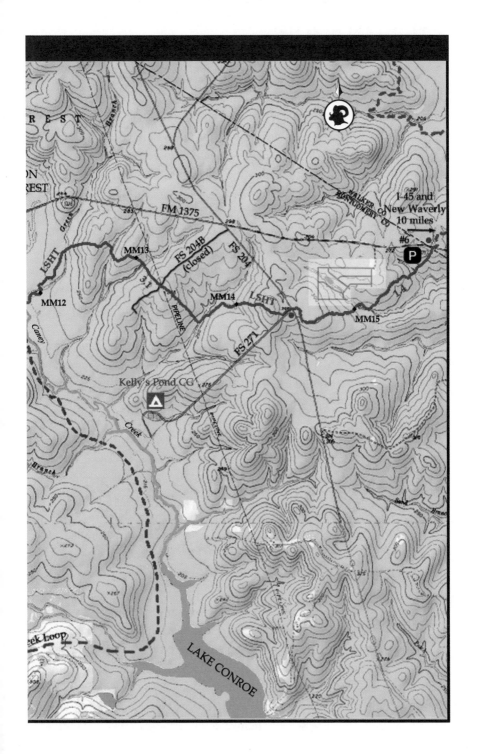

may be some standing water in this area. As you begin to cross a maze of normally dry gullies at mile 9.8, a small

Water ⟁ pond ⟁⟁⟁⟁ may be visible on the left just before you reach an undefined path that crosses the LSHT.

As you pass **MILE MARKER 10**, keep an eye out for one of the first giant oaks adjacent to the LSHT. An enormous pine on the right also begs attention at mile 10.3. Between mile 10.5 and 10.7, there may be a few open spaces for

Campsite ▲ waterless camping. ▲ At mile 10.9 the trail makes a right turn onto an old woods road before quickly veering left again into the woods. After **MILE MARKER 11**, an old road-bed makes for good tread in a mature pine forest until you reach FS 237/Osborn Road at mile 11.3.

FS 237 is an unstriped paved road with a few parking spots. The LSHT is well marked at this road junction. FM 1375 is located to the left (north) less than a mile up Osborn Road. In the springtime, the scent of honeysuckle will accompany you as you head back into the woods and cross a utilities right-of-way. Do you remember intersecting the Little Lake Creek Loop Trail just after you began hiking at the western terminus? You've now reached its other end at LSHT mile 11.8. The LSHT continues straight, while the orange-blazed Little Lake Creek Loop heads right and back toward the LSHT's western terminus (reached in 18.5 miles). A designated primitive campsite is located 0.5

Campsite Ⓐ mile down the Little Lake Creek Loop trail. Ⓐ

Water ⟁ You immediately head down to Caney Creek, ⟁⟁ which normally flows in cool weather on its way to Lake Conroe, only 2 miles downstream. Quiet hikers may walk up on wood ducks enjoying the clean creek water. In this hardwood bottomland grows a variety of vegetation: dwarf palmettos, oaks, and hanging vines. A lone mature pine rises a hundred feet above scattered river cane, one of three temperate bamboo species native to North America. These flat seasonal bottomlands can also be covered with thick

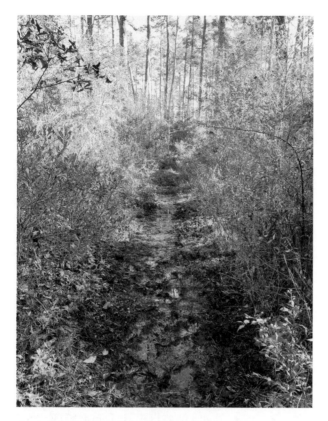

A muddy stretch of the LSHT in Section 2, common during rainy periods

grasses that obscure the LSHT. Luckily, trail markers are plentiful. This low area is usually muddy, but in dry times there are several potential campsites ▲ along the creek.

▲ Campsite

MILE MARKER 12 is in a picturesque grove of large oaks hung with Spanish moss, which is not actually a true moss but a bromeliad, or relative of the pineapple. This moss does not typically harm its host trees and provides a home for insects, snakes, and some species of bats. In the past, American Indians used Spanish moss for clothing and medicinal purposes, while pioneers used it to caulk cabins and stuff saddle blankets. At mile 12.2 you cross a dry drainage that has the potential to hold quite a bit of runoff during wet weather. Look for more palmettos, thorny vines, river cane, and the shortest-lived oak species, the water oak (*Quercus nigra*). With lifespans of 60–80 years, the large water oaks here are nearing old age.

Near mile 12.5 the trail rises up out of the swampy bottomland onto a pine-dominated upland. The path continues to climb until it crosses a heavily used ATV track at the top of a hill. A small creek that usually has clear, flowing water 🚰 is crossed soon afterward. Reach **MILE MARKER 13** just before you cross another creek—this one usually dry—on a small, leaning bridge. Soon top a gentle rise in an open forest of mature pines.

Water 🚰

A good gravel road (FS 204B; closed to traffic) crosses the trail perpendicular to a pipeline right-of-way at mile 13.3. At mile 13.7 and 13.8, cross two small creeks that are dry most of the time. You may spot an old trail marker a hundred feet before the actual **MILE MARKER 14**, attached to an oak tree. At mile 14.1 cross a well-used ATV track, and at mile 14.2 ascend to a uniquely picturesque hilltop view (elevation 300'), from which you can see a dirt road ahead and below. At dirt FS 271 (also known as Kelly's Pond Road), there is a bit of impromptu parking; eastbound hikers should follow trail markers left for a short walk down FS 271 to meet FS 204. Directly across FS 204, blazes and signposts then lead hikers back to the LSHT in yaupon-dominated woods. At this junction, 1 mile to the right on FS 271, is Kelly's Pond Hunter Camp. Ⓐ Its eight primitive campsites have picnic tables, fire rings, and a pit toilet (no potable water or electricity; possible fee). The USFS lists all sites along the entire length of Kelly Pond Road as designated (approved) camping during deer-hunting season.

Campsite Ⓐ

At mile 14.5 you cross an abandoned road in mixed woodland. Another sign leads you across a large ATV track at mile 14.6. Soon the trail crosses a smaller bike track as it nears a house. Dogs may begin to bark as you hike past nearby private property, making the wide, flat open areas impractical as campsites. Two more undefined trails intersect the LSHT. The attractive riparian area that follows, with its diversity of hardwood trees, offers a good lunch or break spot.

Just beyond **MILE MARKER 15** are a few open areas peaceful enough to warrant camping, but there is still private property just to the north. ▲ Sand Creek is usually filled with shallow murky water; the trail follows along its banks and then crosses it at mile 15.1. Large loblolly pines appear as the trail heads into a sloping upland. A small, sandy-bottomed creek at mile 15.5 may harbor a trickle of water.

▲ Campsite

Reach FM 1375 at mile 15.7. Ahead is a dirt road that leads to LSHT Trailhead Parking Lot 6. The trail continues into the woods just to the right of the dirt road on the other side of FM 1375. Shortly after you cross the highway, a side trail off the LSHT leads you safely to the parking lot.

SECTION 2 Mileage

MILES W→E	TRAIL POINT	MILES E→W	NOTES
8.7	FM 149, LSHT North Wilderness Trailhead Parking Lot 3	87.7	▬ 🅿
8.9	Junction of trails; left on LSHT	87.5	
9.0	**MILE MARKER 9**	87.4	
9.1	Jeep track; left on LSHT	87.3	
9.3	Junction of trails; left on LSHT; potential camping	87.1	▲
9.8	Pond (hard to see) on left ◊◊◊◊	86.6	◊
10.0	**MILE MARKER 10**	86.4	
10.5	Potential waterless campsites	85.9	▲
10.9	T-junction; right on LSHT	85.5	
11.0	**MILE MARKER 11**	85.4	
11.3	FS 237/Osborn Rd.; trailhead parking	85.1	▬ 🅿

continued on next page

SECTION 2 Mileage

MILES W→E	TRAIL POINT	MILES E→W	NOTES
11.4	Utilities right-of-way	85.0	
11.8	Little Lake Creek Loop (orange-blazed) branches right; designated camping in 0.5 mi	84.6	Ⓐ
11.9	Caney Creek (high volume, good water ♢♢); potential camping	84.5	♢ ▲
12.0	**MILE MARKER 12;** swampy area	84.4	
12.2	Large seasonal drainage	84.2	
12.7	ATV track at top of hill	83.7	
12.8	Creek (low volume, good water 🚰)	83.6	🚰
13.0	**MILE MARKER 13**	83.4	
13.1	Seasonal creek	83.3	
13.3	Pipeline right-of-way; gravel FS 204B	83.1	
13.7	Creek (stagnant water)	82.7	
14.0	**MILE MARKER 14**	82.4	
14.1	ATV track	82.3	
14.2	FS 271 (good dirt road); FS 204 (paved road); Kelly's Pond Hunter Camp 1 mi right on FS 271	82.2	▰ Ⓐ
14.6	ATV track	81.8	
15.0	**MILE MARKER 15;** potential camping; creek (low volume, murky)	81.4	♢ ▲
15.5	Seasonal creek	80.9	
15.8	LSHT Stubblefield Trailhead Parking Lot 6, FM 1375	80.6	▰ 🅿

MILEAGE CHART KEY

▲	Undeveloped campsite or potential camping area	🚰	Water source (seasonal/unrated)
Ⓐ	Designated campsite during hunting season	▰▰▰	Major roads (jeep tracks and logging roads not indicated)
♢	Water source (DROPS-rated)	🅿	Parking area/trailhead

FARM TO MARKET 1375 CROSSING
TO COTTON CREEK CEMETERY ROAD

OVERVIEW

HIGHLIGHTS OF THE CONROE SECTION include a large, view-filled waterfront-camping area on the shore of Lake Conroe, as well as picturesque and peaceful Stubblefield Lake Campground. Both areas offer good wildlife viewing and opportunities to fish. The region between these two highlights also takes hikers into swampy areas that, in wet seasons, can mean wading through calf-deep water for short stretches but can also mean experiencing a lush ecosystem different from any other on the Lone Star Hiking Trail (LSHT). The majority of Section 3, however, is on high-and-dry ground, with well-spaced water sources.

This section ends with a 2-mile road walk that follows peaceful country roads, taking hikers past historic ranches and farms.

Note: The Forest Service (FS) 215 bridge over Stubblefield Lake was severely damaged by Hurricane Harvey in 2017 and remains closed to both vehicle and foot traffic at the time of this writing. The bridge is scheduled for replacement no sooner than August 2020; because it also serves as the LSHT's means of crossing the lake, there is no trail continuity in this section as long as the bridge remains closed. Thru-hikers will need to plan a shuttle around the bridge in the meantime.

TRAIL ACCESS AND PARKING

LSHT Stubblefield Trailhead Parking Lot 6, at LSHT mile 15.8, is located off Farm to Market (FM) 1375, 8.1 miles from I-45. The well-signed parking lot is in the woods just off the highway down a small dirt access road. No water or trash disposal is available.

In addition, there are parking areas on FS 215 (also called Stubblefield Lake Road) at LSHT mile 20.3, on both the east and west sides of the bridge over Stubblefield Lake—again, however, note that this bridge was closed after Hurricane Harvey in 2017 and is slated to be rebuilt no sooner than August 2020. FS 215 can be accessed from FM 1375 a few miles west of LSHT Stubblefield Trailhead Parking Lot 6. The lot on the west side of the bridge, adjacent to Stubblefield Lake Campground, has access to tap water and trash containers.

The wide shoulders along FM 1374 at LSHT mile 23.1 allow cars to safely park along the road during the day but do not provide adequate security for long-term or overnight parking.

SECTION 3 GPS Waypoints	
LSHT Stubblefield Trailhead Parking Lot 6, FM 1375	N30° 31.563' W95° 37.812'
Stubblefield Lake Campground	N30° 33.536' W95° 38.228'
FM 1374, LSHT mile 23.1	N30° 35.253' W95° 36.293'
Intersection of Bath and Ball Roads	N30° 38.040' W95° 35.378'
Beginning of Cotton Creek Cemetery Road	N30° 38.015' W95° 35.218'
End of Cotton Creek Cemetery Road, LSHT mile 28.3	N30° 38.082' W95° 34.964'

SUPPLIES AND ACCOMMODATIONS

New Waverly (population 1,032) lies about 10 miles east of Stubblefield Parking Lot 6 along FM 1375, just east of I-45). New Waverly has no overnight lodging but does offer several combination gas stations/convenience stores, restaurants, an auto-parts store, a library, and a grocery store. From New Waverly, it's 15 miles north on I-45 to the town of **Huntsville,** which offers many options for overnight lodging and all other essential hiker services.

Developed **Stubblefield Lake Campground,** at LSHT mile 19.7, has restrooms with hot showers and tent pads ($15 nightly fee). *Note:* Campsites are available only on a first-come, first-served basis.

WATER

Four reliable sources of water are found in Section 3 directly on the trail: the Lake Conroe shoreline at mile 16.5, a clear-flowing creek at 17.7, Stubblefield Lake Campground at mile 19.7, and Fern Creek at mile 24. Other creeks are seasonal and should not be relied upon during dry weather.

TRAIL DESCRIPTION

Section 3 starts at the LSHT crossing of FM 1375. As the trail reenters the woods here, it quickly intersects a well-signed side trail heading left that leads to LSHT Parking Lot 6; you continue on the main path, gradually climbing through a mature pine forest with a thick undergrowth of yaupon and honeysuckle. Just a few minutes past MILE MARKER 16, the trail heads downhill, toward 22,000-acre Lake Conroe (elevation 201'). ⬡⬡⬡⬡⬡ Completed in 1973, the lake impounds the West Fork of the San Jacinto River. Along the shoreline at mile 16.5, a large open area beneath big pines is a perfect spot for camping, ▲ complete with a nice view and easy access to the lake. At least plan to take a break here; there won't be a better spot until you reach Stubblefield Lake Campground at mile 19.7. Among the trees on the shoreline, you may be able to spot the heart-shaped leaves of the linden (also called the basswood), a large shade tree native to Asia, Europe, and eastern North America. You may also want to keep an eye out for bald eagles, which have been known to nest in this area.

◊ **Water**

▲ **Campsite**

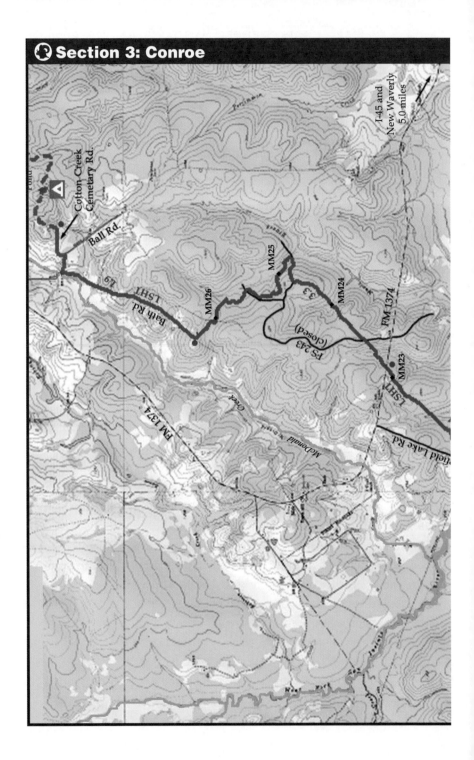

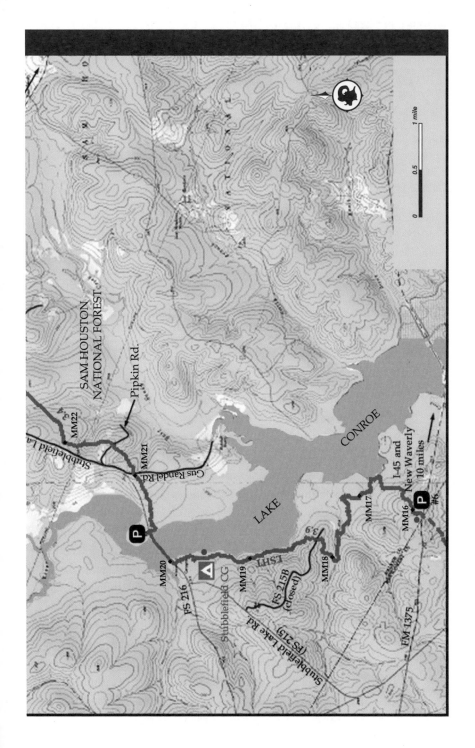

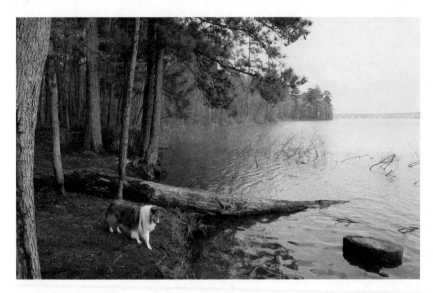

The author's Sheltie heads down to the waters of Lake Conroe for a drink.

As you leave the shoreline, make a left turn to follow the LSHT eastbound. (Remember that if you're hiking from east to west, you'll need to reverse all directions, left and right, in these trail descriptions.) Cross a gully and parallel **Water** 🚰 it until you cross it again at mile 16.8. Although water 🚰 in this gully doesn't usually flow well, it may offer a more appealing (less silt-laden) source compared with Lake Conroe. Brushy yaupon thickets mix here with open, palmetto-filled flats. At **MILE MARKER 17**, the lake is again visible through the trees to the right. There are two decent flat sites **Campsite** ▲ for camping ▲ at miles 17.1 and 17.3. A bridged seasonal creek intersects the LSHT at mile 17.6, which marks entry into an extensive swampy area riddled with honeysuckle thickets. If you find water over the trail, be patient, expect to get a little wet, and make your way around and through it as carefully as you can. The trail soon reaches drier ground again, and you may see some interesting trees and animal life. In particular, the endangered red-cockaded woodpecker may be seen or heard in this area.

At mile 17.7 there is an open place across Quicksand Creek. ◌◌◌◌ This large creek stays next to the LSHT for a bit and contains unusually clear water. Cross this creek at mile 17.9 on a bridge; then cross a seasonal drainage and pass **MILE MARKER 18**. FS 215B (closed to vehicles) intersects the LSHT at mile 18.3. The trail meanders into a jungly area at mile 18.6 but soon reenters a forest of big oaks and pines. Lake Conroe can again be seen off to the right; a few unofficial side trails to the right of the LSHT lead down to the water. **MILE MARKER 19** is located just after the trail dips into a grassy, swampy bottomland sporting profuse gardens of dwarf palmettos and wild dewberry vines. The LSHT heads onward over a series of seasonal creeks in picturesque forests of sweetgum, water oak, hickory, and American holly (*Ilex opaca*), the latter of which reaches its greatest size in these East Texas forests.

◌ **Water**

At mile 19.7 you leave the woods and enter developed Stubblefield Lake Campground. Ⓐ For a nightly fee of $15, the campground offers hikers restrooms with running water, hot showers, potable water, 🚰 and 30 clean sites with picnic tables and tent pads. Stubblefield Lake is now a backwater of Lake Conroe, but it existed as a smaller oxbow lake many years prior to the much larger reservoir. Stubblefield Recreation Area was originally developed by the Civilian Conservation Corps in 1937 as part of President Franklin D. Roosevelt's New Deal.

Ⓐ **Campsite**

🚰 **Water**

From where the LSHT enters Stubblefield Lake Campground, take a right on the paved campground road, and follow it past the picnic pavilion and restroom building; you should see LSHT trail markers leading you in this direction. When you reach FS 215 (Stubblefield Lake Road) and leave the campground behind, take a right on the road and walk over the short road bridge, which is usually host to several people fishing for largemouth bass, crappie, bluegill, and catfish. (*See earlier note regarding the current bridge closure.*) You may also see kayakers and canoeists enjoying this peaceful part of the lake, which is too shallow for motorized boats. This is a good spot along the LSHT to look for alligators, wintering bald eagles, and osprey (fishing eagles). Along this road, you pass **MILE MARKER 20**. After you cross the bridge, a large parking area comes into view on the left, and the LSHT reenters the woods at mile 20.3 through a fenceline on the right. A few minutes later make a sharp left turn, avoiding the old trail that continues straight ahead.

Just past **MILE MARKER 21**, cross unstriped, paved Gus Randel Road, a utilities right-of-way, and then unpaved Pipkin Road. The trail remains well marked. At mile 21.3, cross a seasonal drainage in a pretty area of thick pine, oak, and yaupon. An unmarked trail veers off to the right, and then an ATV track intersects the LSHT. There are some

Campsite ▲ flat spots with room for tents ▲ at mile 21.5 (elevation 290'), but this area is near private property on both sides of the trail. Continue onward past a few more dry gullies on the brushy trail, past a buried pipeline right-of-way, and around several more gullies. A larger intermittent creek, crossed at mile 21.9, may offer some clear, flowing water.

Soon after passing **MILE MARKER 22**, you'll see a deer stand at an open borderline of property boundaries. One of the huge pine trees in this area is a bearing tree used to mark property corners. At mile 22.2 cross a creek that has a stony bottom, something not often seen in East Texas. The trail turns right onto an overgrown jeep track; there are very few trail markers along the old road, but you follow it for a while. Cross another normally dry, rocky-bottomed creek, and then reach a split in the road at mile 22.6. The LSHT takes the left fork, and the woods begin to open up more, even offering a few potential waterless campsites. At mile 22.9, reach a barbwire fence that marks private property, a farmstead, on the left. Try to ignore the trash that seems to accumulate as you pass **MILE MARKER 23**. Very soon you reach the intersection of the LSHT and FM 1374; cross the highway diagonally to the right, and reenter the woods at a hiker gate on the other side of the road. There is no official trailhead parking along FM 1374, though the generous shoulder provides ample room for day parking.

After crossing a few small, seasonal creeks in an open forest, turn left onto a fairly large dirt road at mile 23.5, and follow it for 150 feet; this is FS 243, closed to traffic and used mostly for logging activities. Just past Fern Creek, a small but reliable bridged stream, ⬠⬠⬠⬠ pass **MILE**   ⬠ **Water** **MARKER 24** on a large, fire-scarred pine. Meandering FS 243 is reached again at mile 24.5. Walking down this road, well-spaced trail markers lead you almost 0.3 mile before pointing the way back into the woods on the right side of the road. If you're hiking in the spring, the next few miles make an excellent habitat for nesting woodcocks—robin-size,

Big woods near Mile Marker 23

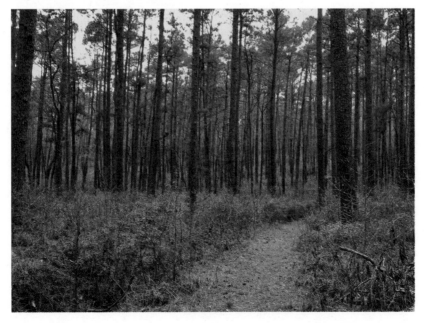

ground-dwelling birds with long, pointed beaks that they use to probe for earthworms.

In this wilder-feeling mixed pine forest, pass **MILE MARKER 25**. A large seasonal drainage, an overgrown logging road, and possible dry camping in some open flats are passed in the next 0.5 mile. At mile 25.5, a large oak tree serves as a hiker bridge over a steep-sided stream. Keep an eye out for red maple trees in the next mile or so; true to their name, they turn a deep scarlet in fall. On the right, several large gullies and creeks come together at mile 25.9. Just a few minutes after passing **MILE MARKER 26**, turn right onto a jeep track. At mile 26.4 make a right onto historic dirt Bath Road. As you walk the next 1.5 miles down Bath Road, you'll pass mile 27, as well as farms (including the historic Harding Ranch, a Texas Century Ranch established in 1850), houses, and horse pastures. You'll also cross MacDonald Creek, which is most likely polluted with livestock runoff.

As you reach the intersection of Bath and Ball Roads at mile 27.9, make a right onto paved Ball Road. LSHT trail markers lead the way past mile 28—there are no mile markers on the road. As you top a small rise, you come to a white gravel road on the right at mile 28.1; this may appear to be a private drive but is, in fact, Cotton Creek Cemetery Road, and you will need to turn left onto it. (*Note:* If you continue on paved Ball Road, which swings to the right here, you may end up walking a long way before you realize your error.) There are only a few trail markers along Cotton Creek Cemetery Road. At mile 28.3, after crossing a second cattle grate, you'll see a green house on the right, followed by a newer brick home. It may feel as if you are walking up their driveway, but soon the road swings to the left and deteriorates to an old, little-used jeep track. A sign lets you know that you're entering the national forest again at mile 28.4, officially the end of Section 3 and the beginning of Section 4.

SECTION 3 Mileage

MILES W→E	TRAIL POINT	MILES E→W	NOTES
15.8	LSHT Stubblefield Trailhead Parking Lot 6, FM 1375	80.6	⇤⇥ 🅿
16.0	**MILE MARKER 16**	80.4	
16.5	Lake Conroe shoreline; ◊◊◊◊◊ large campsite	79.9	◊ ▲
16.8	Creek (medium volume; slow-flowing, semiclear water)	79.6	🚰
17.0	**MILE MARKER 17**	79.4	
17.3	Potential campsite	79.1	▲
17.6	Bridge over seasonal drainage; wetlands	78.8	
17.9	Bridge over Quicksand Creek (medium volume, good water ◊◊◊◊)	78.5	◊
18.0	Cross seasonal drainage; **MILE MARKER 18**	78.4	
18.3	FS 215B (closed to vehicles)	78.1	
19.0	**MILE MARKER 19**	77.4	
19.2	Swampy creek (stagnant water)	77.2	
19.7	Stubblefield Lake Campground	76.7	🚰 Ⓐ
20.0	FS 215/Stubblefield Lake Rd. bridge*; **MILE MARKER 20**	76.4	⇤⇥
20.3	End road walk, reenter woods to right of road	76.1	
21.0	**MILE MARKER 21;** Gus Randel Rd.; utilities right-of-way	75.4	⇤⇥
21.4	ATV track	75.0	
21.5	Potential campsites	74.9	▲
21.7	Fire break or pipeline right-of-way	74.7	
21.9	Seasonal creek	74.5	
22.0	**MILE MARKER 22;** property boundary	74.4	
22.2	Stony-bottomed seasonal creek	74.2	
22.3	Right on old jeep track	74.1	
22.6	Jeep road splits; take left fork	73.8	
23.0	Private farm on left; **MILE MARKER 23**	73.4	
23.1	FM 1374	73.3	⇤⇥
23.5	Left on large dirt road for a few hundred feet	72.9	

Closed; expected to reopen no sooner than August 2020

continued on next page

SECTION 3 Mileage

MILES W→E	TRAIL POINT	MILES E→W	NOTES
24.0	Fern Creek; ◊◊◊◊ **MILE MARKER 24**	72.4	◊
24.5	Right on dirt road for 0.2 mi	71.9	
24.7	Left on LSHT; reenter woods	71.7	
25.0	**MILE MARKER 25**	71.4	
25.2	Large seasonal drainage	71.2	
25.3	Old logging road	71.1	
26.0	**MILE MARKER 26**	70.4	
26.1	Right on jeep track	70.3	
26.4	Right on dirt Bath Road	70.0	▄▄
27.9	Intersection of Bath and Ball Roads; right on Ball Road	68.5	▄▄
28.1	Left on gravel Cotton Creek Cemetery Road	68.3	▄▄
28.3	National-forest property boundary; left on old dirt road	68.1	

MILEAGE CHART KEY

▲ Undeveloped campsite or potential camping area

🚰 Water source (seasonal/unrated)

Ⓐ Designated campsite during hunting season

▬▬▬ Major roads (jeep tracks and logging roads not indicated)

◊ Water source (DROPS-rated)

🅿 Parking area/trailhead

COTTON CREEK CEMETERY ROAD TO EVELYN LANE

OVERVIEW

DESPITE A ROAD WALK AT ITS EASTERN END, the Huntsville
Section of the Lone Star Hiking Trail (LSHT) has a lot to
offer. The walking is pleasant and enjoyable through classic
piney woods. The crossing of Camelia Lake's spillway provides a break from the thick woods, and the LSHT follows
the large creek, Alligator Branch, for more than a mile. A
wide variety of water-loving trees, such as sycamore, and
numerous resident and seasonal bird species can be found
in this area.

Hikers should have little trouble following the trail's
route in Section 4. Only the trail around the west end of
Alligator Branch offers a challenge—even in relatively dry
seasons, expect to get your feet muddy for a few minutes
while walking through this rich swampland.

The LSHT never enters the boundaries of 2,000-acre
Huntsville State Park, but it's close enough to the park to
offer LSHT hikers further recreational opportunities. Pad-
dling the park's lake in a rented canoe, or biking and walking its trails, makes an excellent diversion within a few miles
of the LSHT. Thru-hikers will want to resupply (or at least
grab a hot shower) at Huntsville State Park or along I-45,
where there are several reasonably priced chain motels and
restaurants about 4.5 miles north of the trailhead.

TRAIL ACCESS AND PARKING

There is no parking area on Cotton Creek Cemetery Road,
a narrow forest road at the west end of Section 4 at LSHT
mile 28.3. Neither is there a parking area on paved Evelyn
Lane at the east end of Section 4 at LSHT mile 36.9. That

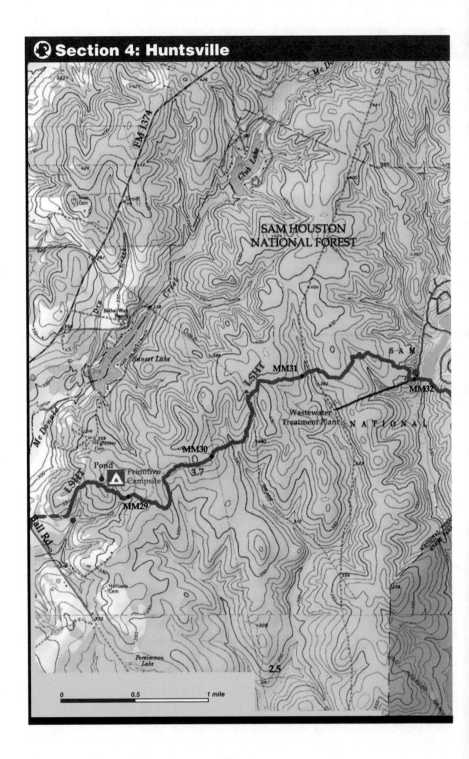

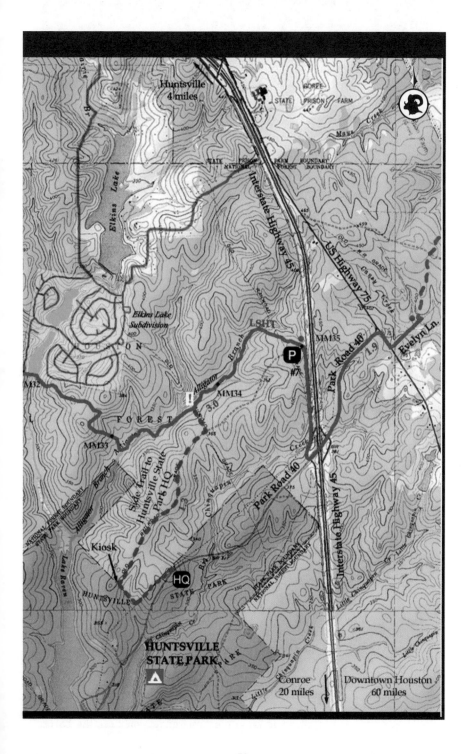

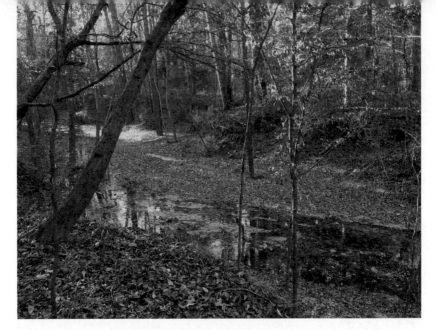

A scenic spot along Alligator Branch in Section 4

said, you could leave a single car or two along the side of these roads during the day for shorter hiking excursions. In addition, there is no official parking lot or trailhead in Elkins Lake Subdivision, but you could park a car at the end of Camelia Drive for day hikes.

To access the LSHT at mile 32 (where it crosses through the outskirts of the Elkins Lake Subdivision) from the I-45 feeder road, about 5 miles south of the city of Huntsville or about 2 miles north of the Huntsville State Park exit off of I-45, turn onto Augusta Drive headed west into the Elkins Lake Subdivision. Go 0.5 mile to the intersection of Augusta Drive and Greenbriar Street. Turn left on Greenbriar, and go 1.1 miles to River Oaks Drive. Turn right onto River Oaks Drive, then left on West Green Briar Drive, and then veer left onto Camelia Drive. Camelia ends at a circular drive where you will see a small road at the head of the circle.

To get to the LSHT, you'll either drive or walk a few feet up this small drive and turn right on the unstriped, paved road that leads to the wastewater treatment facility. Just after you cross the cattle grate, you'll see the LSHT heading off into the woods westbound. The eastbound LSHT follows the unstriped road you just came up and crosses over the Camelia Lake spillway.

The only official parking lot in Section 4 is along the LSHT at mile 35, where **LSHT Huntsville Trailhead Parking Lot 7** is located, on the west side of I-45 along the two-way feeder road adjacent to the interstate. There is no water here, but tap water is available at Huntsville State Park, about 2 miles south of this parking lot. LSHT Parking Lot 7 is a little smaller than the other official lots but is well signed and visible from the feeder road.

SECTION 4 GPS Waypoints	
End of Cotton Creek Cemetery Road, LSHT mile 28.3	N30° 38.082' W95° 34.964'
Camelia Lake Spillway	N30° 38.848' W95° 32.505'
LSHT Huntsville Trailhead Parking Lot 7, along I-45	N30° 38.995' W95° 30.636'
Turn under I-45 onto Park Road 40	N30° 38.372' W95° 30.600'
Junction of Park Road 40 and TX 75	N30° 39.101' W95° 30.127'
End of road walk on Evelyn Lane, mile 36.9	N30° 39.172' W95° 29.833'

SUPPLIES AND ACCOMMODATIONS

Huntsville State Park, near the east end of Section 4, is a good stopover within walking distance of the LSHT that will appeal to thru-hikers. To reach the park, turn right (east) onto Park Road 40 at the intersection of the I-45 feeder road and Park Road 40 at LSHT mile 35.6, and go about 1 mile to reach the park entry gate; a $5 entrance fee is required. Hikers can also access the park via a 1.3-mile unofficial side trail accessed at LSHT mile 33.8.

Farther into the park (another 0.5–1 mile), a developed campground has sites availale for $15 (water only) or $20 per night (water and electricity); the park entrance fee also applies. Camping reservations by phone or online (see

Appendix A, page 155) are recommended. The park provides potable water, restrooms with running water and hot showers, beverage vending machines, a seasonal camp store (open 9:30 a.m.–4:30 p.m. Friday–Sunday, with extended hours in the summer), and boat rentals. For those interested in overnight parking, there is a $2 daily fee per vehicle; check with the park for other parking restrictions, such as location and time limits.

The park doesn't accept or hold hiker packages, but hikers who are willing/able to travel into town can send resupply packages to the U.S. Post Office in Huntsville (936-295-4362) at the following address: **[Hiker Name], c/o General Delivery, 3190 TX 30 W., Huntsville, TX 77340.** Be sure to include a note on the front of your package explaining when you plan to pick it up, e.g., "Hold for LSHT Hiker; ETA 1/16/2020."

Huntsville (population 38,548), one of Texas's oldest towns, is located about 6 miles north of LSHT Trailhead Parking Lot 7. Of course, a town this size has nearly every accommodation or resupply option a hiker could need. Home to Sam Houston State University, Huntsville also hosts several interesting attractions, including the Sam Houston Homestead and Memorial Museum, the Sam Houston Statue and Visitor Center, and the Prison Museum. It's 2 miles north of where you come out at the trailhead on I-45 to a combination convenience store/gas station, located on the feeder road. It's 4.5 miles north of the trailhead to a large freeway exit at FM 1374 East, where there are several restaurants, hotels, and gas stations with ATMs. If you need additional services, continue north, following the signs, to reach downtown Huntsville, at the intersection of TX 75 and TX 30, about 6 miles north of LSHT Trailhead Parking Lot 7.

New Waverly (population 1,032) is about 8 miles south of the intersection of Park Road 40 and TX 75. The town has no overnight lodging but does have several combination gas stations/convenience stores, restaurants, an animal clinic, an auto-parts store, a library, and a grocery store.

WATER

Two reliable water sources grace Section 4: a fairly clear, wild pond at mile 28.9 and the large, clear waters of **Alligator Branch** between miles 33.3 and 34.3 (access to the creek is easiest at mile 33.3). **Camelia Lake,** crossed midway through this section at mile 32.1, is not recommended as a water source due to constant runoff from the lawns and streets that surround it. A 1-mile detour at LSHT mile 35.6, right onto Park Road 40, will bring you to the entrance gate of Huntsville State Park, where potable water and cold sodas in vending machines are available.

TRAIL DESCRIPTION

As Cotton Creek Cemetery Road transitions to an even smaller dirt road and enters Sam Houston National Forest at LSHT mile 28.4, you officially enter Section 4. Follow this old dirt road to an intersection with a very small logging track on the right at mile 28.8. Turn right, walking over a dirt mound, and follow the LSHT trail markers into the woods. (Remember that if you're hiking westbound, you'll need to reverse all directions, left and right, in these trail descriptions.) In less than 0.3 mile, the trail passes along the shores of a pond ⚪⚪⚪ that offers a few tent pads and a fire ring at a designated backpacker's site on its easternmost side. Ⓐ The pond's waters are an acceptable drinking source for those carrying water-treatment equipment. Reach **MILE MARKER 29** just after the pond.

⚪ Water

Ⓐ Campsite

At mile 29.4, the sharp-eyed hiker may spot an 8-foot-high game fence that parallels the LSHT on the right through the heavy brush and trees. Cross a seasonal drainage and watch for an old wooden milepost, which is located at current mile 29.5. You may notice a few large oaks and pine trees nearby. Just after crossing a pipeline right-of-way where the game fence is clearly in view to the right, you'll pass **MILE MARKER 30**. As you near mile 30.4, heavy brush may begin to close in on the trail. A tornado passed through these woods more than a decade ago, leaving openings in the tree canopy where mature trees were knocked down by high winds. This is one way that nature gives young plants and trees a chance to grow in thick forests. Watch for Southern red cedar and American holly in this area.

Don't miss the left turn at mile 30.6. Follow an old barbwire-fence line on a pine needle–covered trail that

A beautiful swamp at mile 33.1 near Alligator Branch

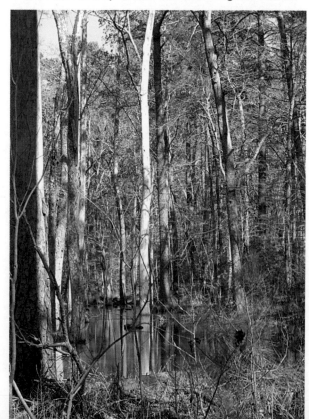

makes for more open, pleasant walking. In fact, waterless camping ▲ is possible on either side of the trail at mile 30.7. Watch for **MILE MARKER 31** between the crossings of two seasonal drainages just before you arrive at another, brushier pipeline right-of-way. At mile 31.3, among old pine trees, you may pick up the sounds of a nearby downstream wastewater treatment facility. It is hidden by the trees but can be noisy. Pass a small stream at mile 31.5. This area is frequented by feral pigs; evidence of their presence can be seen along the sides of the trail as rooted-up clumps of dirt and plant matter, along with occasional mud wallows.

▲ Campsite

Cross another seasonal drainage, and climb a knoll under big trees. You should spot several houses in Elkins Lake Subdivision at mile 31.9. Another 50 yards of walking brings you to **MILE MARKER 32** and, soon after, a small road. Turn left on this unstriped, paved road (the wastewater treatment facility is down this road to the right). Walk on the road downhill, toward the lake and over a cattle grate. Hikers used to be able to get water from the exterior taps of the small brick pumphouse you will now pass by, but water is unavailable there at the time of this writing.

You've now reached an interesting hiker obstacle: the Camelia Lake Dam. The LSHT crosses directly over the dam, where water trickles across a flat, mossy spillway. This spillway can be very slippery, so take your time crossing it. *Note:* There is no better way to continue on the LSHT without walking through the neighborhood's confusing streets or fording the stream in the thick woods below the spillway.

After crossing the spillway, head up the rise through the hiker gates. Veer to the right after the second hiker gate, and walk over a dirt hump intended to keep ATVs and bikes off of the trail. Continue directly into the woods— *do not continue into the neighborhood.* Continued local support for the LSHT relies on hikers respectfully crossing through privately owned areas such as Elkins Lake; for this reason, hikers shouldn't rely on this neighborhood as a source of trail information or water. Come prepared with your own resources; filtering water out of Camelia Lake is not a good option.

The LSHT heads uphill after leaving Camelia Lake as it begins a 3-mile stretch of uninterrupted woods before reaching I-45. You may continue to see houses and hear dogs to the left of the trail for the next 0.5 mile. The first waterless **Campsite ▲** campsites ▲ can be found at mile 32.6 in an open forest of mature pines. Continue to follow a pretty ridge rich in upland hardwood species such as sassafras, flowering dogwood, rusty blackhaw, and post oak mixed with loblolly and shortleaf pine. Invasive nandina plants grow throughout these woods, no doubt having been spread by birds feeding in nearby human landscapes.

After **MILE MARKER 33**, the trail passes a mountain bike trail and heads downhill into the bottomlands of Alligator Branch. A few extraordinarily large specimens of dwarf palmetto rise overhead as you pass. On quiet days, beautifully colored wood ducks may be in the swamps that you'll cross at mile 33.2. Expect to get your feet very muddy, if not soaked, for a short stretch. And watch for trees ringed at the base by busy beavers, animals that were all but extinct in this region 30 years ago.

Water ◊ Alligator Branch ◊◊◊◊ flows year-round with clear spring-fed water over pure white sands that are common along the larger waterways of East Texas. In warmer months, you may even discover a small swimming (or at least soaking) hole along this fine creek. Despite its name, it's very unlikely that you'll spot an American alligator here, though this is one of the finest sections of the LSHT for bird-watching.

At mile 33.3, there is a pretty spot under the canopy of a holly growing on the creek bank, one of the best places to collect water if you need it. Small natural clearings along the creek and in the pines just ahead are the best camping spots to be had until you reenter the woods after the I-45 road walk. Continue to parallel Alligator Branch, passing several isolated oxbows (filled with brown, swampy water) that serve as important refuges for seasonal waterfowl.

You may now begin to hear the distant roar of the interstate. At mile 33.8, the LSHT intersects an old logging rail bed; this overgrown, elevated pathway now serves as part of an unmaintained and unmarked shortcut trail for hikers to reach designated camping and other amenities at Huntsville State Park. A simple signpost marked only with a red exclamation point is currently the only indication of this unofficial shortcut to the park. To follow it, turn right off the LSHT, and head down the old rail bed for about 0.1 mile before turning right onto narrow, brushy Forest Service Road 286 (closed to vehicles). The state park boundary is marked by a kiosk 1.3 miles from the LSHT. From the kiosk, turn left and go 0.3 mile to reach park headquarters, where you'll pay the required daily entry fee. For an LSHT hiker heading to Huntsville State Park, this unofficial side path saves miles of road walking; by following all state park rules, you ensure that the park system will continue to allow LSHT hikers access to the park via this shortcut.

Just before passing **MILE MARKER 34**, the LSHT rejoins Alligator Branch, whose banks have now grown quite steep and high. Look for the mottled white bark of sycamore trees adjacent to the trail through this area. Cross a deep, V-notched ravine on a footbridge at mile 34.2. Veer to the right at the trail junction at mile 34.7; westbound hikers should watch carefully here, as there are few trail markers in sight. **MILE MARKER 35** is reached just before the trail leaves the woods and arrives at the small LSHT Huntsville Trailhead Parking Lot 7, located on the I-45 feeder road.

Now begin a 2-mile road walk that takes you under I-45 and back to public lands where the LSHT runs on toward Cleveland: from LSHT Trailhead Parking Lot 7, turn right on the feeder road, and walk along the west side of I-45 for 0.6 mile to a stop sign. Turn left at the stop sign onto Park Road 40, which leads underneath the freeway. (If you turn right here, it's a little more than a mile along the park road before you reach the entrance to Huntsville State Park, beyond which is developed camping, a small seasonal camp store, potable water, vending machines, and hot showers; entrance and camping fees are charged.) Walk under the overpass and continue straight on Park Road 40 for 1 mile to a stop sign, passing mile 36 somewhere along the way.

At the stop sign, turn right on TX 75 and walk 0.1 mile to Evelyn Lane, an unstriped paved road on the left. Turn left onto Evelyn Lane, walk past a house with a pond and fence on the left, and continue 0.2 mile to a gated driveway. Just to the right of the blue metal gate, on the left side of Evelyn Lane near a barbwire fence, the LSHT heads into the woods with plenty of trail markers showing the way. As you enter the woods, you're between LSHT miles 36.9 and 37.0, and at the unceremonious eastern end of Section 4.

SECTION 4 Mileage

MILES W→E	TRAIL POINT	MILES E→W	NOTES
28.3	National-forest property boundary; left on old dirt road	68.1	
28.4	Leave old dirt road; right over hump into woods on LSHT	68.0	
28.9	Pond; ◊◊◊ designated camping	67.5	◊ Ⓐ
29.0	**MILE MARKER 29**	67.4	
29.5	Seasonal drainage	66.9	
30.0	Cross pipeline right-of-way; **MILE MARKER 30**	66.4	
30.7	Enter open area with potential camping; seasonal drainage	65.7	▲

SECTION 4 Mileage			
MILES W→E	TRAIL POINT	MILES E→W	NOTES
31.0	Seasonal drainage; **MILE MARKER 31**	65.4	
31.3	Elkins Lake water-treatment plant visible	65.1	
31.5	Seasonal stream	64.9	
32.0	**MILE MARKER 32;** Elkins Lake subdivision; left on paved road	64.4	▭
32.1	Cross Camelia Lake spillway (likely polluted)	64.3	
32.6	Seasonal drainage; potential waterless campsites in pine forest	63.8	▲
33.0	**MILE MARKER 33**	63.4	
33.1	Cross tributary of Alligator Branch; enter swamplands	63.3	
33.3	Alligator Branch (low flow, clear, spring-fed ⬦⬦⬦⬦)	63.1	⬦ ▲
33.8	Cross old rail bed; shortcut 1.6 mi to Huntsville State Park to right	62.6	Ⓐ 🅿
34.0	**MILE MARKER 34**	62.4	
34.7	Junction of trails; right on LSHT	61.7	
35.0	**MILE MARKER 35;** I-45; LSHT Huntsville Trailhead Parking Lot 7; right on I-45 feeder road	61.4	▭ 🅿
35.6	Left on Park Road 40; continue under I-45 (Huntsville State Park is about 1 mile right on PR 40)	60.8	▭
36.6	Right on TX 75	59.8	▭
36.7	Left on Evelyn Lane	59.7	▭
36.9	Left on LSHT, to the right of blue metal gate	59.5	

MILEAGE CHART KEY

▲	Undeveloped campsite or potential camping area	🚰	Water source (seasonal/unrated)
Ⓐ	Designated campsite during hunting season	▭▭	Major roads (jeep tracks and logging roads not indicated)
⬦	Water source (DROPS-rated)	🅿	Parking area/trailhead

EVELYN LANE TO FOUR NOTCH TRAILHEAD
ON FOREST SERVICE ROAD 213

OVERVIEW

ONLY 4.8 MILES OF SECTION 5 are routed in the woods. However, the remaining 3.4 miles of road walking are mostly enjoyable, as they follow the scenic country lane named Four Notch Road. Water can be an issue for long-distance or overnight hikers through this section, but the flip side of that concern is a trail nearly free of the intermittent mud and standing water that can be a hindrance in other sections.

In the few places where leaves or brush has obscured the trail, the LSHT remains well marked by aluminum blazes. A subtle transition from thick piney woods and swampy bottomlands to more-open pine–oak highlands occurs as the LSHT reaches the eastern half of Section 5. Tree species, such as Southern magnolia, rarely encountered to the west of Section 5, are seen in the Phelps Section.

TRAIL ACCESS AND PARKING

There is no parking area on Evelyn Lane, at the west end of Section 5 at LSHT mile 36.9, although there is room for a car to squeeze onto the dirt shoulder. **Four Notch Trailhead Parking Lot 8,** on Forest Service (FS) Road 213, is 0.2 mile off Four Notch Road at the east end of Section 5. There is no water at this large lot, but there is a covered picnic pavilion and trash dumpster serving the adjacent Four Notch Hunter Camp. To reach Parking Lot 8 from the intersection of TX 75 and Farm to Market (FM) 2296 about 5 miles north of New Waverly, go north for 4.2 miles on FM 2296; then turn right and head east for 2.3 miles on Four Notch Road. At FS 213, go left (north) for 0.2 mile to reach the Four Notch parking lot and trailhead, at LSHT mile 45.1.

SECTION 5 GPS Waypoints	
End of road walk on Evelyn Lane, mile 36.9	N30° 39.172' W95° 29.833'
FM 2296 at LSHT mile 42.0	N30° 39.359' W95° 27.547'
Intersection of FM 2296 and Four Notch Road, mile 42.6	N30° 39.765' W95° 27.262'
LSHT Four Notch Trailhead Parking Lot 8, mile 45.1	N30° 38.769' W95° 25.396'

SUPPLIES AND ACCOMMODATIONS

Huntsville and **New Waverly,** both at the west end of Section 5, offer resupply within a reasonable distance of the LSHT. Only Huntsville offers overnight lodging. See Section 4 (page 73) for additional information. The east end of Section 5 along Four Notch Road at LSHT Trailhead Parking Lot 8 is in a remote area; neither supplies nor accommodations are located near the trail.

WATER

Unfortunately, Section 5 is one of the driest on the LSHT. In rainy periods or prolonged wet seasons, there are several seasonal drainages throughout this section that may harbor trailside water. In most normal–dry seasons, however, you should plan carefully to carry all the water you need to traverse this section. Along the road walk on Four Notch Road, between miles 42.6 and 45.1, there are two creeks, one of which is the large and reliable Winters Bayou. Their proximity to the road and local farms may deter hikers.

TRAIL DESCRIPTION

As you leave Evelyn Lane and the 2-mile road walk at the end of Section 4, the LSHT heads back into the woods, just to the right of a blue metal gate near a barbwire fence, and quickly passes **MILE MARKER 37**. At mile 37.4, cross a small

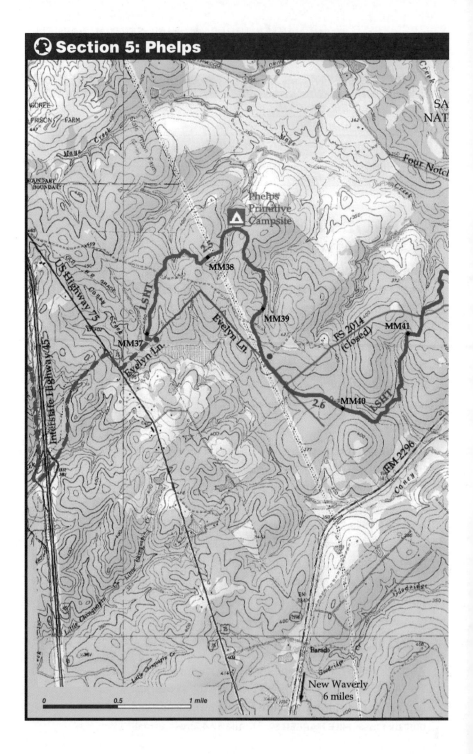

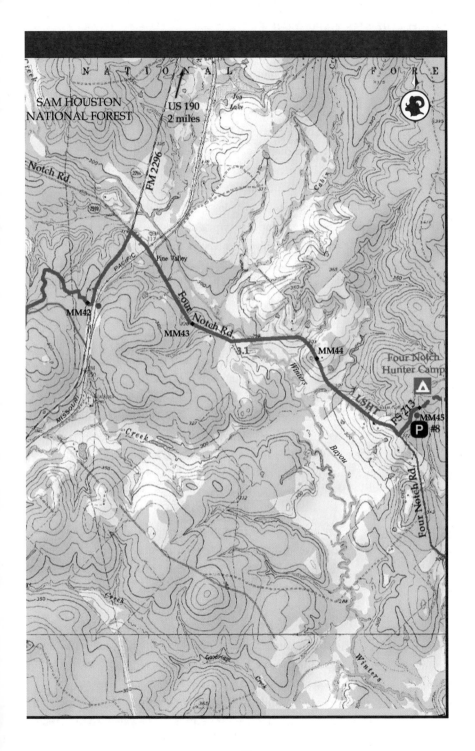

seasonal drainage and an old abandoned logging road. The trail crosses another steep-sided seasonal drainage, traverses a young pine forest, and begins to zigzag before crossing a good jeep road. (Remember that if you're hiking westbound, you need to reverse all directions, left and right, in these trail descriptions.)

In an open, grassy area beneath mature pine trees, pass **MILE MARKER 38** just before reaching a utilities right-of-way. A waterless camp ▲ could be set up here. Cross a small hiker bridge over a creek that may harbor a trickle or a puddle at mile 38.2. Approved for camping during deer-hunting season, Phelps Primitive Campsite offers a fire pit and room for four or five tents at mile 38.3. Ⓐ Ascend a hill, and cross a grassy logging road and old wooden milepost 38 at current mile 38.6. Another seasonal drainage follows soon after. Watch for the numerous holly trees that grow to the right of the trail in this area, which feels as if it is seldom walked. There's even a good (waterless) campsite ▲ under a holly on the left at mile 38.9. Pass **MILE MARKER 39** a few minutes before you turn onto an overgrown track to the left. Enter an area of shortleaf pine and large hardwood trees, including white oak, Southern red oak, black hickory, and sassafras. This is a nice spot for a break.

At mile 39.3 you pass through a hiker gate and turn left onto a gravel road near the power lines; this is actually Evelyn Lane again, though it's gravel here. Walk on this road until mile 39.7, where you turn left back into the woods by a hiker sign and a house where dogs may be running loose.

As you reenter the peace of the woods, the LSHT passes through a young pine forest along a wide corridor. Just after an old logging road, pass **MILE MARKER 40**. A bridge spans a seasonal creek that usually has water running in it at mile 40.4. Watch for large white oaks through here; these long-lived trees produce valuable wood that's

Campsite ▲

Campsite Ⓐ

Campsite ▲

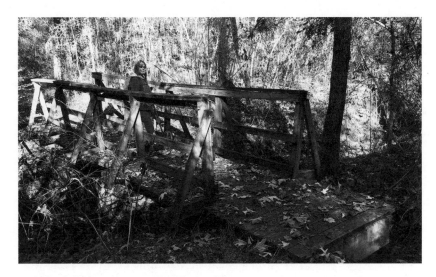

A hiker bridge crosses a seasonal creek.

often used for making furniture. A large creek at mile 40.5 may contain stagnant water in wet seasons, followed by another seasonal creek. Then pass another of the few remaining original wooden mileposts, this one indicating mile 41 though it's located at current mile 40.8. Soon reach modern **MILE MARKER 41** (elevation 395'), which leads into a section of mature open pine forest near a boundary with private land. Cross a large gravel road at mile 41.2. East-bound hikers pass one of the first noticeable evergreen Southern magnolia trees (*Magnolia grandiflora*) on the left. Also called the bull bay, the tree's large, thick, fragrant blossoms evolved before bees existed and are shaped spe-cifically to be pollinated by beetles.

Cross an old logging road at mile 41.6, followed by a seasonal drainage and pipeline right-of-way. The trail may be hard to see underfoot as you near **MILE MARKER 42**, so watch for the well-spaced trail markers in the trees at eye level. Don't forget, though, to look down occasion-ally; beautiful mushrooms, such as cinnabar chanterelles, are commonly seen alongside the trail here. You may also notice some houses off to the left.

Soon reach FM 2296 and begin a road walk by turning left and walking on the side of this highway for about 0.5 mile. Reach signed Four Notch Road at mile 42.6, and turn right onto this unstriped, paved road, directly across from the intersection of the larger FM 2929 and FM 2296. At mile 42.8, still on the road walk, cross the railroad tracks and continue straight ahead on Four Notch Road. You soon **Water** cross a creek that should have running water in it; if you're thirsty, follow this creek a little upstream and off the road to find a safe place to collect and treat its water. **MILE MARKER 43** is visible along the road in a tree.

At mile 43.7 you pass a house where some large farm dogs may come out to bark at you. Then cross another **Water** large creek with running water, Winters Bayou. You may be thirsty enough to search for a good place to filter water, despite the nearby pastures. **MILE MARKER 44** is hard to see but is passed as you come up a hill and follow a curve in the road. Open farmland allows the eye to roam on either

The route briefly returns to gravel Evelyn Lane at mile 39.3.

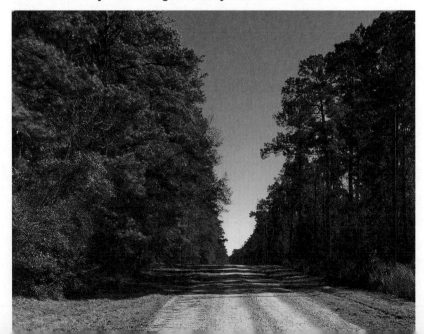

side of this little country lane. Except for the occasional dog or two, this is a peaceful, scenic road walk.

At mile 44.9 a double-blazed set of trail markers directs you to turn left down dirt FS 213. **MILE MARKER 45** is not visible, but you'll know you've just passed it when you arrive at the oversize parking lot at the end of this section, at mile 45.1. This is LSHT Four Notch Trailhead Parking Lot 8, which does double duty as designated Four Notch Hunter Camp. Ⓐ Dumpsters, a picnic shelter, and a trailhead bulletin board are located at this wayside; there is no water, however. This site is the location of the old Four Notch fire tower; you may see some of its foundation. As you leave this parking lot and reenter the woods, the 3-mile Phelps road walk ends, and you enter Section 6.

Ⓐ **Campsite**

SECTION 5 Mileage

MILES W→E	TRAIL POINT	MILES E→W	NOTES
36.9	Left into woods right of blue metal gate	59.5	⚎
37.0	**MILE MARKER 37**	59.4	
37.4	Seasonal drainage; abandoned logging road	59.0	
37.6	Large, sandy-bottomed gully	58.8	
37.7	Steep-sided seasonal drainage	58.7	
37.8	Jeep track	58.6	
38.0	**MILE MARKER 38**; open, grassy area; potential campsite	58.4	▲
38.2	Bridge over small seasonal creek (stagnant water)	58.2	
38.3	Phelps Primitive Campsite	58.1	Ⓐ
38.4	Grass-covered logging road	58.0	
38.6	Old wooden milepost 38	57.8	
38.7	Seasonal drainage	57.7	
38.9	Potential campsite	57.5	▲
39.0	**MILE MARKER 39**	57.4	
39.1	Left on jeep track across power line	57.3	

continued on next page

SECTION 5 Mileage

MILES W→E	TRAIL POINT	MILES E→W	NOTES
39.3	Hiker gate; left onto gravel Evelyn Lane	57.1	▬▬
39.7	Reenter woods on left	56.7	
40.0	Old logging road; **MILE MARKER 40**	56.4	
40.4	Bridged seasonal creek (small amount of flowing water)	56.0	
40.5	Large seasonal creek (stagnant water)	55.9	
40.6	Seasonal creek	55.8	
41.0	**MILE MARKER 41**	55.4	
41.2	Gravel road	55.2	
41.6	Old logging road	54.8	
41.7	Seasonal drainage	54.7	
41.9	Pipeline crossing	54.5	
42.0	**MILE MARKER 42;** left on FM 2296	54.4	▬▬
42.6	Right on Four Notch Road	53.8	▬▬
42.8	Cross railroad tracks; continue on Four Notch Road	53.6	
43.0	Creek (low volume 🚰); **MILE MARKER 43** along Four Notch Road	53.4	🚰
43.7	Cross Winters Bayou (high volume 🚰) on Four Notch Road bridge (*note:* pastures nearby)	52.7	🚰
44.0	**MILE MARKER 44;** Four Notch Road	52.4	
44.9	Left on dirt FS 213	51.5	▬▬
45.0	**MILE MARKER 45,** FS 213	51.4	
45.1	LSHT Four Notch Trailhead Parking Lot 8; reenter woods on right	51.3	▬▬ 🅿️ Ⓐ

MILEAGE CHART KEY

▲	Undeveloped campsite or potential camping area	🚰	Water source (seasonal/unrated)
Ⓐ	Designated campsite during hunting season	▬▬	Major roads (jeep tracks and logging roads not indicated)
🌢	Water source (DROPS-rated)	🅿️	Parking area/trailhead

**FOUR NOTCH ROAD TO JUNCTION OF
FOREST SERVICE ROADS 207 AND 202**

OVERVIEW

THE FOUR NOTCH LOOP AREA was devastated by a pine bark beetle infestation in the early 1980s. The U.S. Forest Service (USFS) cut, burned, and replanted the damaged forests between 1982 and 1987; today it's difficult for even the most observant hiker to discern where the natural, wild forest transitions to the replanted areas. Despite the large segments of newer growth, the heart of this section is nearly devoid of usable roads and thus retains a wild, remote feel and a diversity of forest types.

The well-maintained, 10-mile Four Notch Loop Trail, of which the main LSHT is a part, offers an excellent opportunity for weekend loop hikes with easy trail access at LSHT Trailhead Parking Lot 8. Boswell Creek, located in a beautiful hardwood bottomland, is large enough to offer swimming holes. In most seasons it's easy to find a place to hop from one sandy bank to another; this creek can present an insurmountable obstacle during heavy rains, however. The Four Notch Section is popular with Boy Scouts and other hiking groups, but there's plenty of space for everyone in its wilderness.

The only negative aspect of Section 6 is the 2.7-mile road walk on its eastern end for those wanting to connect with Section 7 on foot. The walk is fairly pleasant, though, following USFS roads through mostly wooded land.

TRAIL ACCESS AND PARKING

To reach **LSHT Four Notch Trailhead Parking Lot 8,** at the west end of Section 6 (LSHT mile 45.1), start at the intersection of TX 75 and Farm to Market (FM) 2296,

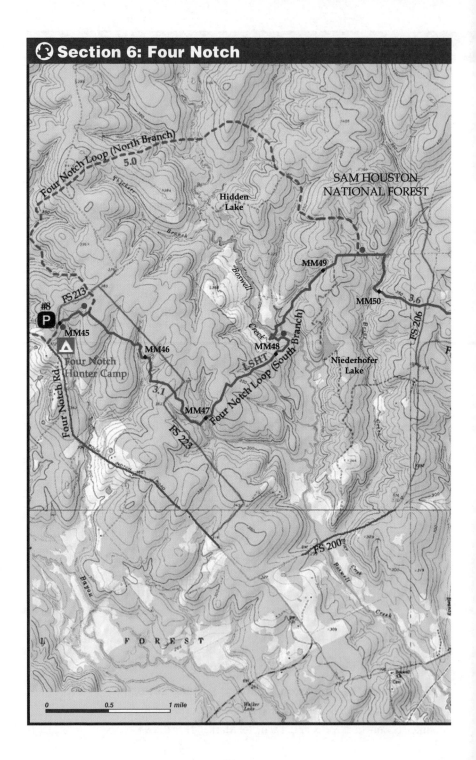

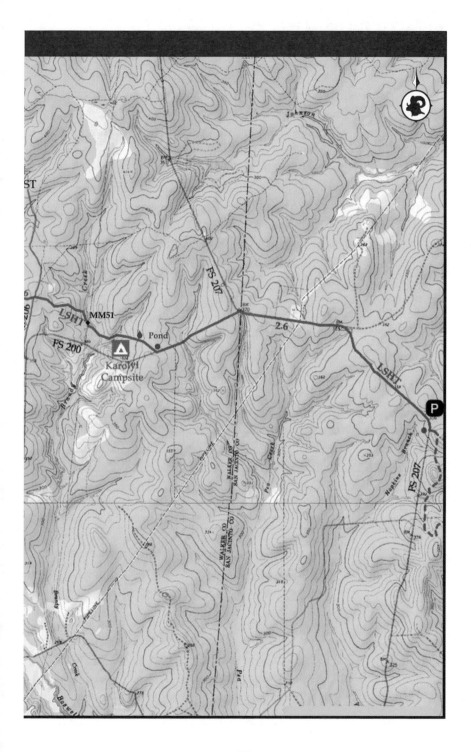

about 5 miles north of New Waverly, and go north for 4.2 miles on FM 2296; then turn right and head east 2.3 miles on Four Notch Road. At Forest Service (FS) Road 213, go left (north) 0.2 mile to reach the Four Notch parking lot and trailhead at LSHT mile 45.1. Dumpsters and a covered picnic pavilion accompany the designated hunter camp here, but note that there is no water at this trailhead.

To reach the east end of Section 6, at the junction of FS 207 and FS 202 (LSHT mile 54.4), proceed to the tiny hamlet of Evergreen at the intersection of FM 945 and TX 150, about 15 miles east of New Waverly. From this intersection in Evergreen, head west toward New Waverly on TX 150 for 0.25 mile, and turn right onto FS 202/John Warren Road (note that this road may be poorly signed). Follow FS 202 for about 7.5 miles until you reach the intersection with FS 207. The LSHT enters the woods to the right of where these two dirt roads intersect. *Note:* No water or trash disposal is available at this trailhead.

SECTION 6 GPS Waypoints	
LSHT Four Notch Trailhead Parking Lot 8, mile 45.1	N30° 38.769' W95° 25.396'
West junction with Four Notch Loop Trail	N30° 38.837' W95° 25.117'
Boswell Creek, mile 48.2	N30° 38.085' W95° 24.219'
East junction with Four Notch Loop Trail	N30° 39.220' W95° 23.016'
Intersection of FS 207 and FS 202, mile 54.4	N30° 37.999' W95° 19.172'

SUPPLIES AND ACCOMMODATIONS

Both the west and east ends of Section 6 are located in remote areas. The town of **New Waverly** (population 1,032) is 5 miles north of the intersection of TX 75 and FM 2296. New Waverly has no overnight lodging but does offer several combination gas stations/convenience stores, restaurants, a post office, an animal clinic, an auto-parts store, a library, and a grocery store. The closest overnight accommodations, as well as a large selection of other services, can be found along I-45 in and around the town of **Huntsville** (see Section 4, page 73, for more information).

WATER

Unlike the Phelps Section, the Four Notch Section is blessed with abundant water sources. Overnight hikers should be able to camp near water at Boswell Creek or at the wild pond at mile 51.5. In wet periods, the seasonal creeks also harbor water. Because of the sandy soils in this region, the creeks tend to run clear, not muddy.

TRAIL DESCRIPTION

From LSHT Four Notch Trailhead Parking Lot 8 and its designated hunter camp, Ⓐ head into the woods, following the trail and LSHT markers visible on the right as you entered the parking lot at mile 45.1. (Remember that if you're hiking westbound, you'll need to reverse all directions, left and right, in these trail descriptions.) After crossing a small seasonal drainage, you soon reach the signed junction of the LSHT and Four Notch Loop Trail at mile 45.4—the loop heads left, following red-blazed trail markers, while the main LSHT turns right. Although this description focuses on the main route, feel free to follow either branch, as they meet again 4 miles down the main branch. (The left-hand fork offers great hiking through some of the most beautiful forests on the LSHT, also crosses Boswell Creek, and is a little longer—closer to 5 miles— before it meets up with the main LSHT.)

At mile 45.7, you cross a deep drainage (elevation 350') that may harbor a trickle or a stagnant pool, followed quickly by a logging road. You may spot some large black

Ⓐ **Campsite**

tupelos (blackgums) as well as Southern magnolia trees, which are much more common on the eastern half of the LSHT. Cross another usually dry, steep-banked creek at mile 45.9. The trail intersects and briefly follows a faint logging road just before reaching **MILE MARKER 46**. Over the next 0.5 mile, you cross several seasonal drainages before reaching a large, open area near unpaved FS 223. Although

Campsite ▲ there's room for several tents here, ▲ be aware that this site can attract car campers and hunters. As you pass the campfire pit, hang a right onto a wide path. Reach a good dirt road, jog slightly to the left, and proceed through an opening that looks like an impromptu parking spot. Continue straight ahead, following trail markers.

Campsite ▲ A more secluded (but waterless) camping spot ▲ is on the right at mile 46.7. You'll cross several typical sea-

Water ◊ sonal creeks, including one at **MILE MARKER 47**. ◊◊ A few large oaks grow in this hardwood forest. Cross two old logging roads—take a sharp left on the first one—before reaching a big, open flat at mile 47.4 where several tents

Campsite ▲ could be set up (this site is also waterless). ▲ At mile 47.5, you join the old logging road again and follow it for

Campsite ▲ some time. More waterless camping ▲ is available at mile 47.6 just before the old road splits—follow the left fork.

Water ◊ Cross another seasonal creek, ◊ and follow the road as it jogs left and then meets another old road.

Pine forests give way to beautiful hardwood bottomland where you pass **MILE MARKER 48**. Beaver activity is

Water ◊ evident along the banks of Boswell Creek, ◊◊◊◊ at mile 48.2. Thru-hikers can celebrate the halfway mark here!

Campsite ▲ Backcountry campsites ▲ are dispersed throughout the woods in this area. The creek's clear waters flow year-round and offer a good water source; in fact, you can spot fish in its waters.

Frequent flooding has washed out all trail bridges over Boswell Creek, so hikers must find their own way

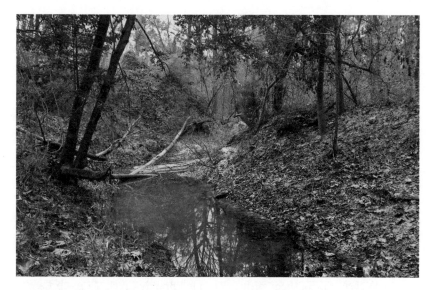

Unbridged Boswell Creek is picturesque and relatively easy to ford, except after heavy rains.

across the creek. In normal-to-dry seasons, the ford should be a quick hop across, but if it has been raining heavily, *this high-banked creek may be extremely hazardous to cross,* so turn back if you find conditions too dangerous for a ford.

After you cross Boswell Creek, turn right and follow it for a short stroll before turning and heading off into the woods. Cross a tributary of the creek, and pause to admire a unique landscape where ferns grow under giant pines. At mile 48.5, a fence becomes visible on the left. After you cross yet another seasonal drainage and pass **MILE MARKER 49**, intersect the Four Notch Loop Trail at its east end at LSHT mile 49.4 at a well-signed junction. This junction makes a nice spot for resting or eating lunch, surrounded by upland hardwood forest dominated by white oak and winged elms. About 40 yards southeast of this junction is a natural pond where you can see large black tupelos and palmettos. Cross a small drainage and traverse a noticeable rise in the land.

At mile 49.7, you meet up with and follow Briar
Water Creek, a large, unbridged, intermittent stream that usually runs with clear water—and is potentially dangerous
after heavy rains. Pass **MILE MARKER 50**, cross a small seasonal drainage among red maples, and then cross FS 206,
a good dirt road. There is some informal parking on either
side of the road here. The trail through this area is sometimes open but usually brushy; as has been the case over
the past few miles, you may sometimes find it necessary
to use the trail markers for visual navigation as you walk.

Just before a pipeline right-of-way, you pass **MILE
MARKER 51**. Oaks and mature pine trees mix throughout
this riparian woodland, making a pleasant spot for a break.
After crossing several unbridged seasonal drainages, one
Water of them fairly steep-sided Brandy Creek, reach Karolyi
Campsite Primitive Campsite at mile 51.4. This designated camp
is named for Bela Karolyi, famous for coaching Olympic
gymnasts (his training facility is located about a mile away
as the crow flies). The camp has a fire ring, tent sites, and a
trail register. A pond just ahead and on the left, at mile 51.5,
Water serves as a treatable water source. Though it can be
a picturesque spot in the fall, briars and brush can make
Campsite finding a good campsite near the pond challenging.
The water here is colored like strong tea by tannins, natural
chemical substances (harmless to ingest in small quanti-
ties) that leach out from leaves and pine needles. You may
find that the water in this pond is not as clear and appealing
as that in the trailside pond in the Huntsville Section.

Cross an old logging road at mile 51.7; then quickly
reach FS 200 (note that there is no room to park a car where
the trail comes out on this road). To begin the 2.7-mile road
walk, turn left on this gravel road and follow it 0.7 mile.
Water Along the way, pass a fairly large creek that should harbor
running water. **MILE MARKERS 52, 53, AND 54**, which used
to be located along the road walk, have likely succumbed

to vandalism, storm damage, or logging and have not been replaced. At mile 52.4, reach a stop sign and turn right onto FS 207, which is also a good gravel road. Walk past a gas-processing plant and beside a young pine forest near mile 53. Keep an eye out for roadrunners, which like to frequent these piney-woods roads. Continue past a small dirt road that heads off to the left; you curve to the right on the main road and pass a picturesque ranch on the left.

The junction of FS 207 and FS 202 is located at mile 54.4. Here, where FS 202 branches off to the left, the point where the LSHT heads back into the woods is well signed and easy to see. There is no parking area here, but there is room for several cars to pull off on the road shoulder. This is the end of Section 6 and the beginning of the seventh section, Big Woods.

SECTION 6 Mileage

MILES W→E	TRAIL POINT	MILES E→W	NOTES
45.1	LSHT Four Notch Trailhead Parking Lot 8; Four Notch Hunter Camp; reenter woods on right	51.3	⊟ 🅿 Ⓐ
45.4	Junction with Four Notch Loop Trail (red-blazed); main LSHT turns right	51.0	
45.7	Deep seasonal drainage; logging road	50.7	
45.9	Seasonal creek	50.5	
46.0	Faint logging road; **MILE MARKER 46**	50.4	
46.2	Seasonal creek	50.2	
46.5	Hunter camp on dirt FS 223; potential campsites	49.9	▲
46.7	Potential camping on right; parallel seasonal drainage on right	49.7	▲
46.8	Large seasonal creek	49.6	
47.0	**MILE MARKER 47**; seasonal creek ◊◊	49.4	◊
47.1	Left on old logging road	49.3	
47.2	Cross logging road	49.2	
47.4	Large, open flat; potential camping	49.0	▲

continued on next page

SECTION 6 Mileage

MILES W→E	TRAIL POINT	MILES E→W	NOTES
47.5	Right on old logging road	48.9	
47.6	Large, open flat; potential camping; seasonal creek ◊	48.8	◊ ▲
47.8	Junction of old logging roads	48.6	
48.0	**MILE MARKER 48**	48.4	
48.2	Boswell Creek (high volume, good water ◊◊◊◊); camping	48.2	◊ ▲
48.7	Seasonal drainage	47.7	
49.0	**MILE MARKER 49**	47.4	
49.4	Junction with Four Notch Loop Trail (red-blazed)	47.0	
49.5	Small seasonal drainage; hill	46.9	
49.7	Briar Creek (seasonal flow; good water 🚰)	46.7	🚰
50.0	**MILE MARKER 50**	46.4	
50.4	Cross FS 206	46.0	▬
51.0	**MILE MARKER 51**; pipeline right-of-way	45.4	
51.1	Large, seasonal Brandy Creek ◊	45.3	◊
51.4	Karolyi Primitive Campsite	45.0	Ⓐ
51.5	Pond on left (dark, tannin-colored water ◊◊◊); camping	44.9	◊ ▲
51.7	Left on gravel FS 200 (no parking)	44.7	▬
51.9	Creek (low volume, good water 🚰) along FS 200	44.5	🚰
52.4	Right on gravel FS 207 at stop sign	44.0	▬
53.0	Gas-processing plant	43.4	
54.4	Junction of FS 207 and 202; reenter woods	42.0	▬ 🅿

MILEAGE CHART KEY

▲	Undeveloped campsite or potential camping area	🚰	Water source (seasonal/unrated)
Ⓐ	Designated campsite during hunting season	▬▬▬	Major roads (jeep tracks and logging roads not indicated)
◊	Water source (DROPS-rated)	🅿	Parking area/trailhead

**JUNCTION OF FOREST SERVICE ROADS 207
AND 202 TO IRA DENSON ROAD**

OVERVIEW

WOODS, WOODS, AND MORE WOODS! The Big Woods Section lives up to its name, leading the hiker through many uninterrupted miles of typical East Texas forests. These pine and oak forests are drained by numerous fern-lined seasonal creeks that feed the watershed of Winters Bayou, itself a major tributary of the San Jacinto River. *Reliable* water sources are scarce, however. During warm or dry seasons, hikers should plan to carry in all the water needed for hiking and camping.

Human development is also relatively sparse in the Big Woods Section of the LSHT. The trail skirts private property that abuts the Sam Houston National Forest in a few places. Small-scale road-building and logging may be visible in these areas, but no major roads or housing developments are located anywhere along the 8.4-mile route.

Likewise, no notable trail obstacles are present—the extended muddy areas and swamps present in so many of the other sections are virtually nonexistent here. Creeks and drainages are easy to cross in all but the worst weather conditions. The trail continues to be well marked. Provided that you're careful to carry in drinking water, Section 7 offers numerous quiet spots to pitch a tent and enjoy the peace of the big woods.

TRAIL ACCESS AND PARKING

To reach the west end of Section 7, at the junction of Forest Service (FS) Roads 207 and 202 (LSHT mile 54.4), proceed to the tiny hamlet of Evergreen, at the intersection of Farm to Market (FM) 945 and TX 150, about 15 miles

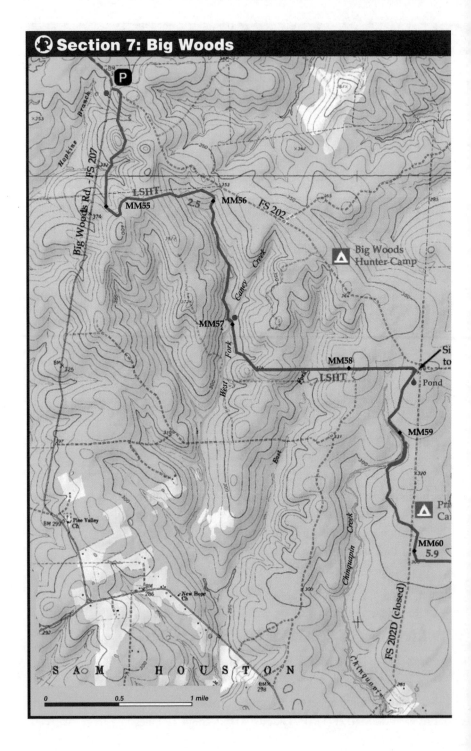

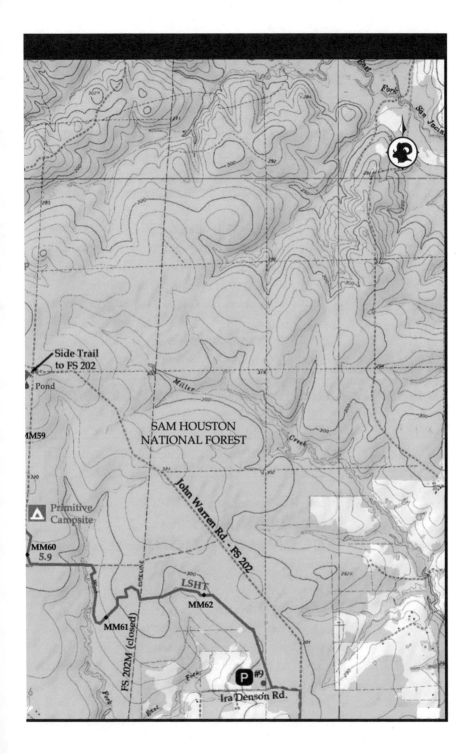

east of New Waverly. From this intersection in Evergreen, head west toward New Waverly on TX 150 for 0.25 mile, and turn right onto FS 202/John Warren Road (note that this road may be poorly signed). Follow FS 202 for about 7.5 miles until you reach the intersection with FS 207. The LSHT enters the woods to the right of where these two dirt roads intersect. *Note:* No water or trash disposal is available at this trailhead.

To reach the east end of Section 7, at **LSHT Big Woods Trailhead Parking Lot 9** (LSHT mile 62.8), follow the directions above through the second sentence. Follow FS 202 for 1.7 miles to the intersection with Ira Denson Road, possibly not well marked, on the left. Take a left onto Ira Denson Road, and go 0.2 mile to Parking Lot 9, on the right side of the road. *Note:* No water or trash disposal is available at this trailhead.

SECTION 7 GPS Waypoints

Intersection of FS 207 and FS 202, mile 54.4	N30° 37.999' W95° 19.172'
West Fork Caney Creek, mile 56.9	N30° 37.258' W95° 18.493'
Side trail to FS 202, mile 58.5	N30° 36.419' W95° 17.123'
LSHT Big Woods Trailhead Parking Lot 9, Ira Denson Rd.	N30° 34.656' W95° 15.464'

SUPPLIES AND ACCOMMODATIONS

The west end of Section 7 is located in a remote area and therefore has no supplies or accommodations close by. The east end of Section 7 is also remote, but just ahead, along the next section's road walk, hikers pass through **Evergreen,** a tiny hamlet of private residences, a Baptist church, and a community center that generously offers hikers tap water.

From Evergreen, it's about 9 miles east to Coldspring (population 853) on TX 150. Coldspring has no

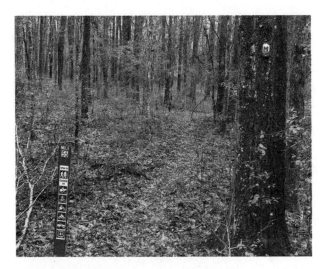

A view down the trail from Mile Marker 55

overnight lodging but does have a local diner, a barbecue restaurant, a post office, a dollar store, gas stations, and a large grocery store. The larger, full-service town of **Shepherd** (population 2,319), 11 miles southeast of Coldspring along US 59, has several motels.

WATER

Section 7 harbors several large seasonal (that is, intermittent) creeks and streams—during dry periods, do *not* expect to find water in this section. Even in wet seasons, if you plan to camp in the Big Woods Section, carry all the water you need to make a waterless camp. The best spot to find water is a small forest pond in the woods, 50 yards off the trail at mile 58.6.

TRAIL DESCRIPTION

The junction of FS 207 with FS 202 is located at LSHT mile 54.4. Here, where FS 202 branches off to the left, the entry of the LSHT back into the woods is well signed and easy to see. Cross a deep seasonal drainage at mile 54.6, and enter a fairly open area where you could set up a waterless camp **Campsite ▲** **▲** on either side of the trail in a mixed forest. Pass several seasonal drainages before you reach **MILE MARKER 55**.

Note: Several tools show that Mile 54 measures 1.2 miles—this is probably due to an inaccurate measurement of the miles along the road walk at the end of Section 6 when the marker was installed. Other mile markers along the LSHT are also slightly short or long, but this guidebook ignores these inaccuracies to avoid confusion.

Cross another small drainage before coming out into an appealing open area in a pine forest. The trail is in good condition as you continue, crossing a twin set of seasonal drainages at mile 55.3. Next, cross an old sunken road and a clearing off to the left where you could put up a **Campsite ▲** tent. **▲** Recross the old road at mile 55.5, and then cross a seasonal drainage twice at mile 55.8. Just as you reach a drainage on the left, pass **MILE MARKER 56**. (Remember that if you're hiking westbound, you need to reverse all directions, left and right, in these trail descriptions.)

Again, dip into and out of that same seasonal drainage a few more times and begin to parallel it at mile 56.5. This is the intermittent West Fork of Caney Creek, which you eventually cross at mile 56.9 and where you have an opportunity to collect water, if there's any to be had. As you climb out of this drainage, the trail turns along a barbwire-fence line on the right. Soon after, reach a marked property boundary where private land abuts national forest. You may see evidence of small-scale road-building on the private land along the LSHT here.

Pass **MILE MARKER 57** in a young pine forest where wild pigs often root up the soil along the trail. Cross a U-shaped, sandy-bottomed seasonal drainage at mile 57.7 in a pretty area. Just after an uphill jaunt, pass **MILE MARKER**

58 in a mixed woodland that's home to some big oaks. In a pinch, you may be able to find a small camping spot off to the left here. ▲

▲ Campsite

Cross an old roadbed and then twice cross a steep seasonal drainage filled with ferns at mile 58.2. Reach a large sign at a sharp right turn in the trail at mile 58.5. A short side trail, in the direction of the arrow of the lower sign reading FS 202/WARREN RD., offers a 0.1-mile shortcut to FS 202 and a small parking pad that could be used by day hikers in this section.

As you turn to the right, look for a small pond ◊◊◊◊ hidden a few hundred feet into the woods on the left side of the trail—this is one of the few reliable water sources in this section, and it also offers potential camping on its far side. ▲ Watch for the giant oak tree to the left of the trail at mile 58.8 and a nearby open area that could be used as a waterless campsite. ▲ Feral pigs often tear up the soils in this area; they are not native to the US but are descendants of domestic pigs that escaped or were released from settlements dating back as far as the first Europeans in East Texas.

◊ Water

▲ Campsite

▲ Campsite

Pass **MILE MARKER 59** and dip into seasonal, fern-lined Chinquapin Creek; there are some possible tent sites in the woods to the left of the trail here. ▲ At mile 59.4 enter a young pine forest and jungly thickets where the woods are reclaiming old logged areas. Cross a seasonal drainage, and then cross a small gravel road (FS 202D; closed to traffic) at a right-trending diagonal at mile 59.8. A small blue triangle points to a designated primitive campsite 100 yards to the left (north) along FS 202D. Ⓐ

▲ Campsite

Ⓐ Campsite

MILE MARKER 60 is soon followed by a set of small drainages and an old logging road where you'll turn left and pass through a young pine forest. If it has been raining, expect to get your feet wet crossing the large, sandy, seasonal creek at mile 60.4. Just after the creek, the LSHT makes a hard right turn. Cross several smaller drainages before you reach a junction of trails at mile 60.9. Follow the LSHT left, and soon pass **MILE MARKER 61**. At mile 61.4, reach an open area at a junction of old logging roads where

Campsite ▲ you could set up a waterless camp. ▲

The trail gradually veers right before taking a sharp left at mile 61.5. Yaupon thickets at mile 61.7 can be quite muddy after rain. Make a right turn at mile 61.9 to meet up with an old logging track. The trail zigs and zags before passing **MILE MARKER 62**.

Pass a fence corner and post at mile 62.4. More bulldozer activity may be evident around this property boundary off to the right. A small opening to the left of the trail

A very well-signed trail junction

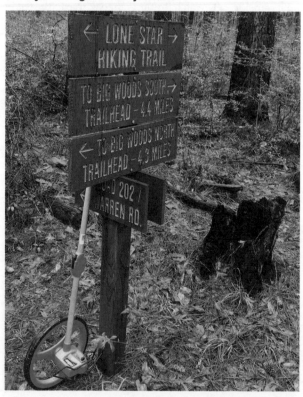

could serve as a waterless camp at 62.5. ▲ In a homog-   **▲ Campsite**
enous young pine forest, walk down the wide and pleasant
trail to mile 62.8 and the end of Section 7, at LSHT Big
Woods Trailhead Parking Lot 9 at dirt Ira Denson Road.
Ahead is the beginning of Section 8—and the longest road
walk on the LSHT.

SECTION 7 Mileage

MILES W→E	TRAIL POINT	MILES E→W	NOTES
54.4	Junction of FS 207 and 202; reenter woods	42.0	▬ 🅿
54.6	Deep seasonal drainage; potential camping	41.8	▲
55.0	Series of seasonal drainages; **MILE MARKER 55**	41.4	
55.3	Twin seasonal drainages	41.1	
55.4	Cross sunken road twice; potential camping	41.0	▲
55.8	Cross seasonal drainage twice (stagnant water)	40.6	
56.0	**MILE MARKER 56**; cross drainage to the left in 0.1 mi	40.4	
56.2	Seasonal drainage; West Fork Caney Creek (trickle of water)	40.2	
56.9	West Fork Caney Creek (low volume, clear water 🚰); property boundary	39.5	🚰
57.0	**MILE MARKER 57**	39.4	
57.7	Shallow seasonal drainage; larger U-shaped drainage	38.7	
58.0	**MILE MARKER 58**; potential camping	38.4	▲
58.1	Old road bed	38.3	
58.2	Cross fern-lined seasonal drainage twice	38.2	
58.5	Signed 0.1-mi side trail to FS 202	37.9	
58.6	Pond off-trail 50 yd left; ◊◊◊◊ potential camping	37.8	◊ ▲
58.8	Large oak tree; potential camping	37.6	▲
59.0	**MILE MARKER 59**	37.4	
59.1	Fern-lined Chinquapin Creek; potential camping	37.3	▲
59.5	Seasonal drainage	36.9	
59.8	Primitive campsite; FS 202D (closed to vehicles)	36.6	Ⓐ

continued on next page

SECTION 7 Mileage

MILES W→E	TRAIL POINT	MILES E→W	NOTES
60.0	**MILE MARKER 60;** several small drainages and old logging road	36.4	
60.2	Old jeep track heads uphill to left; follow LSHT straight ahead	36.2	
60.4	Cross large, sandy-bottomed intermittent stream	36.0	
60.6	Cross several small seasonal drainages	35.8	
60.9	Junction of trails; follow LSHT left	35.5	
61.0	**MILE MARKER 61**	35.4	
61.4	Open area at junction of logging roads; potential camping; follow LSHT straight and then right	35.0	▲
61.5	Make a sharp left turn	34.9	
61.7	Deep, brushy, seasonal drainage	34.7	
62.0	**MILE MARKER 62**	34.4	
62.4	Fencepost and corner at property boundary	34.0	
62.5	Potential camping left of trail	33.9	▲
62.8	LSHT Big Woods Trailhead Parking Lot 9; follow LSHT left onto dirt Ira Denson Rd.	33.6	▬ 🅿

MILEAGE CHART KEY

▲	Undeveloped campsite or potential camping area	🚰	Water source (seasonal/unrated)
Ⓐ	Designated campsite during hunting season	▬▬▬	Major roads (jeep tracks and logging roads not indicated)
◊	Water source (DROPS-rated)	🅿	Parking area/trailhead

**IRA DENSON ROAD TO
DOUBLE LAKE RECREATION AREA**

OVERVIEW

THE MAGNOLIA SECTION is long enough to offer a little of everything. The western end consists of a 5-mile road walk on dirt and blacktop roads. Only a short 0.3-mile stretch of the road walk is along a busy highway; the other miles can be sunny but are usually peaceful.

The remaining 7 miles of Section 8 meander through a variety of ecosystems. One of the most amazing of these is a large region of mature evergreen Southern magnolia trees that surround the bottomlands of the East Fork of the San Jacinto River. Here, the LSHT hiker may be surprised to find a rolling landscape and a secret nook in the woods where a small waterfall runs during most seasons.

This section may also throw other surprises at hikers if flooding has occurred recently: bridges, particularly the one over the East Fork, have been known to wash out. As long as the waterways aren't flooded, adventurous hikers can easily ford them if needed.

Double Lake Recreation Area, built in 1937 by the Depression-era Civilian Conservation Corps, offers several diversions from hiking. This 23-acre spring-fed lake is periodically stocked with bass, bluegill, and catfish. There is even a small sandy beach and swimming area that can be enjoyed in warmer months.

TRAIL ACCESS AND PARKING

To reach the west end of Section 8, at **LSHT Big Woods Trailhead Parking Lot 9** (LSHT mile 62.8), begin from the intersection of Farm to Market (FM) 945 and TX 150 in Evergreen. Head west for 0.25 mile, and turn right onto

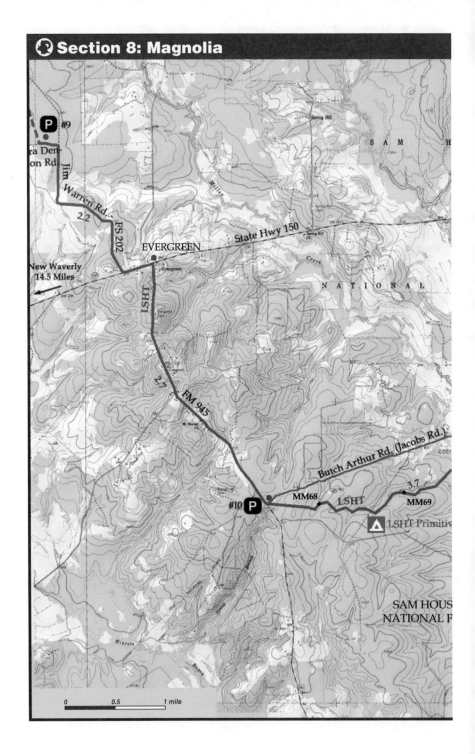

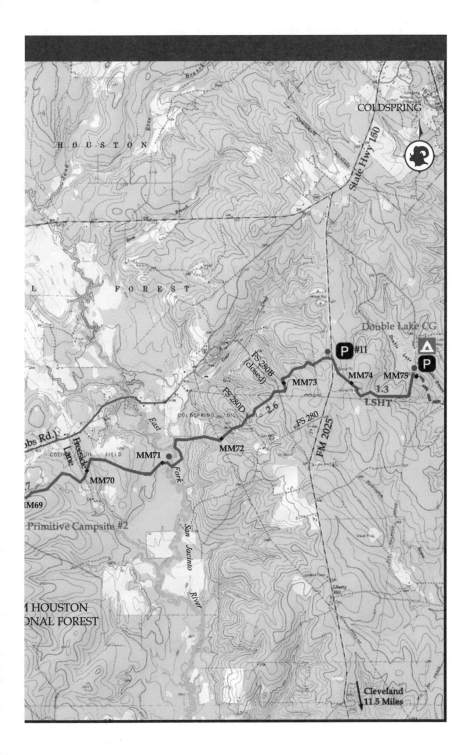

Forest Service (FS) Road 202/John Warren Road (note that this road may be poorly signed). Follow FS 202 for 1.7 miles to the intersection with Ira Denson Road, on the left. Take a left onto Ira Denson Road, and go 0.2 mile to Parking Lot 9, on the right side of the road. *Note:* No water or trash disposal is available at this trailhead.

To reach Double Lake Recreation Area and **LSHT Iron Ore Trailhead Parking Lot 11** from Evergreen, head east for 5.7 miles on TX 150 to Farm to Market (FM) 2025 (or 25 miles east from New Waverly). Turn right (south) onto FM 2025. In 0.4 mile turn left onto Double Lake Park Road to reach the recreation area and its associated parking. (Ask camp hosts about parking a car within the recreation area; there is a $7 daily fee to park here.) Parking Lot 11 is 1.6 miles down FM 2025, or 1.2 miles beyond the entrance to Double Lake Recreation Area.

SECTION 8 GPS Waypoints

Big Woods Trailhead Parking Lot 9, Ira Denson Rd.	N30° 34.656' W95° 15.464'
Intersection of Ira Denson Rd. and FS 202 (John Warren Rd.)	N30° 34.644' W95° 15.281'
Intersection of TX 150 and FM 945, Evergreen	N30° 33.667' W95° 14.335'
LSHT Magnolia Trailhead Parking Lot 10, FM 945 and Butch Arthur Rd. (Jacobs Rd.)	N30° 31.666' W95° 13.207'
LSHT Primitive Campsite 2, mile 68.6	N30° 31.586' W95° 12.110'
Crossing of East Fork of the San Jacinto River	N30° 32.045' W95° 11.074'
LSHT Iron Ore Trailhead Parking Lot 11, FM 2025	N30° 32.886' W95° 08.640'
Double Lake Recreation Area, mile 75.0	N30° 32.759' W95° 07.833'

SUPPLIES AND ACCOMMODATIONS

From Evergreen, at LSHT mile 65.0, it's about 14.5 miles west to **New Waverly** (population 1,032) on TX 150. The town has no overnight lodging but does have several combination gas stations/convenience stores, restaurants, and a grocery store. In the other direction from Evergreen, it's 9 miles east to **Coldspring** (population 853) on TX 150. Like New Waverly, Coldspring has no overnight lodging, but it does have a diner, a barbecue restaurant, a post office, a dollar store, gas stations, and a grocery store. The full-service town of **Shepherd** (population 2,319), 11 miles southeast of Coldspring along US 59, has several motels.

Double Lake Recreation Area has campsites (starting at $20 per night) equipped with picnic tables and campfire rings or a cooking grill. Hot showers, bathrooms with running water, and potable-water taps are located throughout the campground, as are vending machines. A concession stand operates during the warmer months on weekends. During this time of year, camping reservations are recommended (see Appendix A, page 155). These facilities are a few minutes' walk from the LSHT: from mile 75 and the large LSHT sign by the southwest corner of the lake, turn left and head into the campground, which is visible from this spot (the LSHT continues to the right).

WATER

Along the 4.6-mile road walk at the western end of Section 8, water is available only at the intersection of FM 945 and TX 150, where **Evergreen Baptist Church** invites LSHT hikers to use the water taps on the back of its two buildings. There's no need to ask for permission, but please be sure to turn off the water when you've had your fill.

Once you're hiking in the woods, the Magnolia Section has other regular water sources. Many smaller streams dry up in the warmer months, but the East Fork of the San Jacinto River is reliable in any season, although the water here can be extremely silt-laden. Water can also usually be found at a reliable creek crossing at mile 72.2.

At the eastern end of Section 8, potable water is available just 0.2 mile off the LSHT at Double Lake Recreation Area; you can also treat nonpotable water from the lake itself, adjacent to the trail at mile 75.0.

TRAIL DESCRIPTION

From LSHT Trailhead Parking Lot 9, begin this section's 4.6-mile road walk by turning left onto dirt Ira Denson Road where the trail exits the woods into the parking lot. (Remember that if you're hiking westbound, you need to reverse all directions, left and right, in these trail descriptions.) Walk beneath the power lines 0.2 mile to the intersection with dirt FS 202; then turn right onto FS 202 and cross under the power lines again. After 0.5 mile, at LSHT mile 63.5, you'll notice the first farmland along the road. Houses begin to appear soon after.

Reach the intersection of FS 202 (aka John Warren Road) and TX 150 after 2.7 miles on FS 202, at LSHT mile 64.7. Turn left onto TX 150, and walk 0.3 mile past the first road that intersects the highway on the left and a red-brick building on the right. Continue until you reach the intersection of TX 150 and FM 945 at a flashing stoplight at LSHT mile 65.0—this is downtown Evergreen, which offers no services for the road-weary hiker (the larger town of Coldspring is about 8 miles east on TX 150). Be sure, though, to fill your water containers at Evergreen Baptist

Water 🚰 Church, 🚰 located at this intersection; the water taps are located outside on the back side of each of the two buildings on church property. There's no need to ask for permission to get water, but please be considerate and turn off the tap before you leave.

Turn right onto FM 945 at this intersection. LSHT miles 63–67 are passed on this road walk but are not marked along the roads. Pass a cemetery on the left at mile

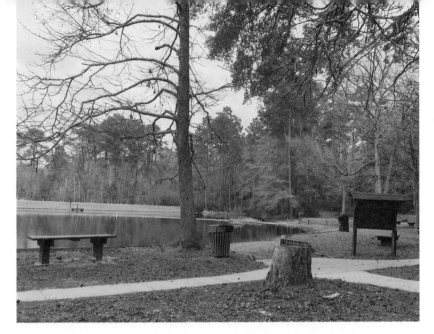

Double Lake Recreation Area is a welcome respite for tired hikers.

65.5, and top a rise at mile 66.0. You pass another cemetery, some houses, and a pretty pond before you reach LSHT mile 67.4 and the intersection of FM 945 and Butch Arthur Road (also known as Jacobs Road). LSHT Magnolia West Trailhead Parking Lot 10 offers shady parking and a trailhead bulletin board near where the trail heads back into the woods at long last. From this point to the eastern terminus, the LSHT has National Recreation Trail status.

Note: The road walk on FM 945 measures a total of 2.7 miles recorded with three different measuring tools, indicating that this LSHT segment is short by 0.3 mile. Technically, then, you're at LSHT mile 67.7, not 67.4, when you reach Parking Lot 10, but to stay consistent with the trail mile markers, this guide ignores that extra 0.3 mile that, unfortunately, your feet cannot.

Now back in the woods, cross a seasonal drainage at mile 67.9 and soon afterward pass **MILE MARKER 68**. Very thick undergrowth prevents camping in a flat area of mature pines. In the spring, watch for the slender wakerobin, also known as the Sabine River wakerobin (*Trillium* *gracile*), a kind of trillium that grows near streams. (Trilliums are three-petaled wildflowers spotted only rarely in Sam Houston National Forest.) Cross a large seasonal drainage on a hiker bridge at mile 68.2. Cross back over the drainage, which may have a bit of water in it during wet seasons, and soon discover a woodland of mature Southern magnolia trees that are this section's namesake. Reach designated LSHT Primitive Campsite 2 at mile 68.6; this backcountry site lies just off the LSHT to the right along an access trail. Several cleared tent sites and a fire ring sit in a large open area, making a convenient site for an overnight stay; you'll need to pack in water, however.

With magnolias shading overhead in every season and honeysuckle blooming profusely in the spring, pass **MILE MARKER 69** in a tree to the left of the trail. Just afterward, at mile 69.1, pass a fence corner on the left. As you notice a larger creek that usually has some water in it, you'll also notice a parcel of private land off to the left—don't collect water or camp in this area. Several large oil and gas fields lie just north of the national forest. At mile 69.3 pass another fence corner and cross the creek, which you'll parallel and cross several times ahead. As an interesting note, you're walking at an elevation of 262 feet above sea level.

At mile 69.8 reach a junction with an ATV track, where you can spot a picturesque horse farm through the trees to the right. Cross dirt Freeside Lane, which leads to the horse farm, and pass **MILE MARKER 70**. The creek you've been crossing multiple times appears again, spanned now by a crooked bridge; this creek drains into the East Fork of the San Jacinto River. Just after you cross the bridge, a sign directs you to make a sharp right-hand turn. The trail follows an old road bed, passing a once-cleared wetland on private property that is now overgrown with young trees; nevertheless, keep an eye out for pileated woodpeckers and barred owls.

Water 🚰

Campsite 🅐

Water 💧

Water 💧

Water 🚰

The LSHT continues to be wide and easy to walk. Large, striking magnolias appear regularly. Wherever they grow, Southern magnolias indicate a subtropical climate.

Reach a hiker gate at mile 70.6. An extremely varied forest emerges at **MILE MARKER 71**; here, wetlands mix with hardwoods, pines, and palmettos. A campsite could be carved out in this location, ▲ which is fairly close to the East Fork of the San Jacinto River ◊◊◊◊◊ (elevation 185'). The hiker bridge over the river was washed out by high water in the early 2000s, but remoteness, expense, and the certainty of future flooding have made replacing it a low priority.

▲ **Campsite**
◊ **Water**

Fording the river when its water levels are normal requires a thigh-deep wade through coffee-colored waters and a slippery ascent up the far bank. We hope a new hiker bridge will be built someday, but for now a small-depth gauge will help you determine the river level. Scout up and down the river for what looks like a good place to cross; sometimes other hikers move large downed trees across the channel to help with the crossing.

Never attempt to cross this river when it's running with a current or flooded—this is one of the largest drainages on the entire LSHT, and it can carry a huge volume of water. If you're confident in your navigational abilities and willing to study online notes and maps, you can make a detour on an unmarked-road walk and bushwhack of about 3 miles between Freeside Lane and FS 280B. For details, including GPS data, photos, and a map, see lonestar trail.org/docs/sanjacdetour.pdf.

Also, unless you're hiking during drought conditions, don't filter drinking water here; just ahead at mile 71.3 is a tributary of the river that normally runs with deep, clear water. ⚱ This tributary is also bridged, as is the next clear, shallow stream at mile 71.6. ⚱ This area supports a variety of hardwood trees and vines that give it the otherworldly

⚱ **Water**

appearance of an ancient jungle. Feral hogs seem to like this area, and it can also be a good place to watch for birds. Begin climbing out of the often-muddy river bottomlands, paralleling an old barbwire fence on the left.

Reach **MILE MARKER 72** in drier pine uplands just before a pipeline right-of-way and jeep track; then head downhill into an interesting rolling area filled with sweet-bay, holly, and magnolia. As you reach the bottom of the draw, find one of the jewels of the LSHT: a beautiful hiker bridge spanning a clear creek with a tiny waterfall.

Water ⬡ ⬡⬡⬡⬡ Here, from August to October, you may also find an uncommon, often overlooked plant called the nodding nixie; this delicate flowering annual is a saprophyte, which feeds off dead and decaying plant material. This is also a good place to look for snakes and frogs.

At mile 72.3 you may notice a flat spot left of the trail that would make a nice campsite cushioned by pine needles.

Campsite ▲ ▲ Cross a good gravel road (FS 280D) and utilities right-of-way at mile 72.4; then cross an old logging road at mile 72.6. At mile 72.8, reach a roadbed and make a sharp right to follow the road, which is now used as service access for a gas pipeline. You'll follow this service road for about 1,000 feet,

A lovely spot along the trail near mile 72

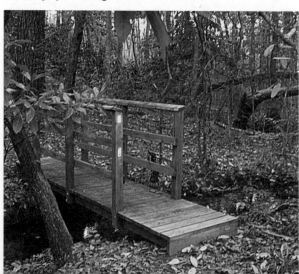

passing over another wide road (FS 280B; closed to traffic) at mile 72.9, before signs lead you back into the woods. Just past **MILE MARKER 73**, make a sharp right. A nice long hiker bridge spans a seasonal gully at mile 73.1. The forest's character has changed to include a wider variety of trees since you crossed the East Fork of the San Jacinto River.

Reach FM 2025 at mile 73.7, and continue straight across this paved road. LSHT Trailhead Parking Lot 11 is located on the east side of the road; a side trail leads hikers to the parking lot at mile 73.9. Cross under utility lines (some open areas here could serve as campsites ▲) and through several hiker gates. Then reach **MILE MARKER 74** (elevation 333'), where thick young undergrowth prevents any further thoughts of camping until you reach the developed campgrounds of Double Lake Recreation Area. Cross an outlying mountain bike path at mile 74.8, just before the LSHT turns into a semipaved surface as it reaches the outskirts of the park's nature trail system.

▲ Campsite

Cross a mountain bike trail at mile 74.9, and continue straight. At **MILE MARKER 75**, break out of the woods by a large LSHT sign, and you'll see spring-fed Double Lake directly ahead. To reach the park's facilities, leave the LSHT here, turn left, and walk along the edge of the lake for a few minutes.

Double Lake Recreation Area has designated campsites Ⓐ (starting at $20 per night) along with hot showers, bathrooms with running water, potable water, 🚰 and vending machines. Canoes and paddleboats can be rented at the seasonal concession stand, which may also sell refreshments and groceries.

Ⓐ Campsite
🚰 Water

The LSHT comes out at the corner of one of the lakes before turning immediately back into the woods—the trail does not continue to Double Lake's facilities. To enter the developed campground, follow the shoreline of the lake toward the buildings visible from the trail. To continue eastbound on the trail into Section 9, make a hard right back into the woods at the large LSHT sign at mile 75 while facing the lake—continuing straight ahead along the top of the lake's dam will take you the wrong way.

SECTION 8 Mileage

MILES W→E	TRAIL POINT	MILES E→W	NOTES
62.8	LSHT Big Woods Trailhead Parking Lot 9; follow LSHT left on dirt Ira Denson Rd.	33.6	⚊ 🅿
63.0	Intersection of Ira Denson Rd. and FS 202	33.4	⚊
64.7	Intersection of FS 202/John Warren Rd. and TX 150; follow LSHT left on TX 150	31.7	⚊
65.0	Intersection of TX 150 and FM 945 in Evergreen; Evergreen Baptist Church (water 🚰); follow LSHT right on FM 945	31.4	⚊ 🚰
65.5	Cemetery on left along FM 945	30.9	
67.4	Intersection of FM 945 and Butch Arthur Rd. (Jacobs Rd.); LSHT Trailhead Parking Lot 10	29.0	⚊ 🅿
67.9	Seasonal drainage	28.5	
68.0	**MILE MARKER 68**	28.4	
68.2	Hiker bridge over large seasonal drainage (low flow, good water 🚰)	28.2	🚰
68.4	Seasonal drainage	28.0	
68.6	LSHT Primitive Campsite 2, to right of trail	27.8	⛺
69.0	**MILE MARKER 69**	27.4	
69.1	Fence corner	27.3	
69.2	Creek (low flow, good water 💧)	27.2	💧
69.3	Fence corner	27.1	
69.4	Creek (low flow, good water 💧)	27.0	💧
69.8	ATV track; horse farm	26.6	
69.9	Freeside Ln. (dirt road)	26.5	
70.0	**MILE MARKER 70**	26.4	
70.1	Hiker bridge over drainage (low flow, good water 🚰)	26.3	🚰

SECTION 8 Mileage

MILES W→E	TRAIL POINT	MILES E→W	NOTES
70.6	Hiker gate; stay straight	25.8	
71.0	Mile Marker 71; straight on LSHT	25.4	
71.1	East Fork of the San Jacinto River ⬤⬤⬤⬤⬤	25.3	⬤
71.3	Hiker bridge over creek (deep, clear water 🚰)	25.1	🚰
71.6	Hiker bridge over stream (shallow, clear water 🚰)	24.8	🚰
72.0	**MILE MARKER 72**; pipeline right-of-way; gravel jeep track	24.4	
72.2	Hiker bridge over creek (shallow, clear water ⬤⬤⬤⬤)	24.2	⬤
72.3	Potential campsite on left	24.1	▲
72.4	Gravel road (FS 280D); utilities right-of-way	24.0	
72.6	Old logging road	23.8	
72.8	Gas-pipeline service road	23.6	
72.9	FS 280B (closed)	23.5	
73.0	**MILE MARKER 73**	23.4	
73.1	Sharp right turn; hiker bridge over seasonal drainage	23.3	
73.7	FM 2025; LSHT Iron Ore Trailhead Parking Lot 11	22.7	▭ 🅿
73.8	Potential camping close to road; utility lines	22.6	▲
73.9	Side trail to LSHT Parking Lot 11	22.5	
74.0	**MILE MARKER 74**	22.4	
74.8	Mountain bike trail	21.6	
74.9	Mountain bike trail	21.5	
75.0	Double Lake Recreation Area; **MILE MARKER 75**	21.4	▭ 🚰 Ⓐ 🅿

MILEAGE CHART KEY

▲	Undeveloped campsite or potential camping area	🚰	Water source (seasonal/unrated)
Ⓐ	Designated campsite during hunting season	▭▭▭	Major roads (jeep tracks and logging roads not indicated)
⬤	Water source (DROPS-rated)	🅿	Parking area/trailhead

DOUBLE LAKE RECREATION AREA TO FM 2666

OVERVIEW

MANY HIKERS FIND THE BIG CREEK SECTION of the LSHT to be the highlight of the entire trail. The most diverse stretch of the 96-mile trail, this section has beautiful forests filled with nearly every species of tree that can be found in the bottomland and upland forests of East Texas.

Double Lake is spring-fed, making it unusually clear and cool for a small lake in this region. The lake feeds one of the major tributaries of Big Creek, which grows increasingly larger and more scenic as it runs toward the 1,420-acre Big Creek Scenic Area. In fact, numerous perennial streams and creeks feed into this protected area, resulting in a lush pine–hardwood forest filled with a variety of flora and fauna. Bird-watchers are particularly enamored with the Big Creek Section.

The LSHT itself remains well marked. The hike covers rolling ground up along the banks of upper Big Creek and down into its bottomlands where wildflowers grow profusely in the spring. There are a few muddy areas, but several are conveniently traversed by boardwalks. Every sizable creek in this section is crossed by a hiker bridge, so there is no worry about having to ford them in rainy weather.

Camping is prohibited within Big Creek Scenic Area. To reduce impact in this beautiful section, plan to camp in either the developed Double Lake Recreation Area campground at mile 75 ($20 nightly fee required) or the semideveloped backcountry site (free) simply named LSHT Primitive Campsite 1 at mile 75.7. Three small loop trails connect to the LSHT within the boundaries of the Big Creek Scenic Area, making this an excellent section for day hiking.

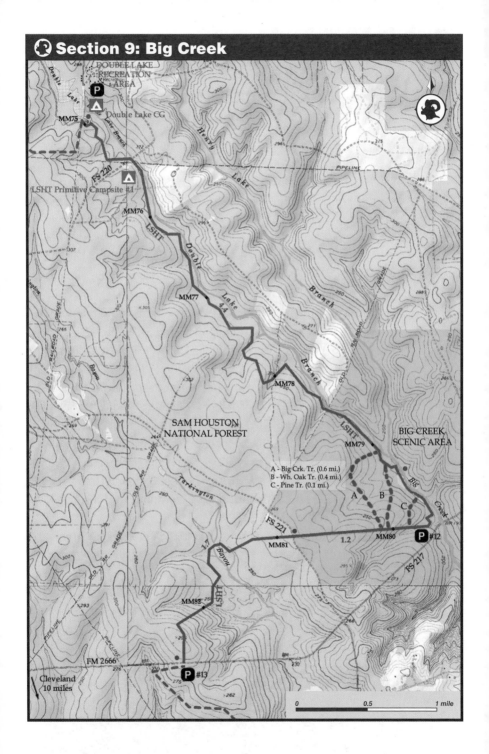

DOUBLE LAKE
RECREATION
AREA

P

Double Lake CG

MM75

Henry Lake Branch

PIPELINE

FS 220

LSHT Primitive Campsite #1

MM76

LSHT

Double Lake 24

MM77

Branch

Branch

MM78

SAM HOUSTON
NATIONAL FOREST

LSHT

MM79

BIG CREEK
SCENIC AREA

A - Big Crk. Tr. (0.6 mi.)
B - Wh. Oak Tr. (0.4 mi.)
C - Pine Tr. (0.1 mi.)

A   B   C

Big Creek

Tarkington

FS 221

MM81

1.2

MM80

P #12

FS 217

1.7

Bayou

MM82

LSHT

PIPELINE

PIPELINE

FM 2666

BM

Cleveland
10 miles

P #13

0   0.5   1 mile

129

TRAIL ACCESS AND PARKING

To reach Double Lake Recreation Area and **LSHT Iron Ore Trailhead Parking Lot 11** from Evergreen, head east for 5.7 miles on TX 150 to Farm to Market (FM) 2025 (or 25 miles east from New Waverly). Turn right (south) onto FM 2025. In 0.4 mile turn left onto Double Lake Park Road to reach the recreation area and its associated parking. (Ask camp hosts about parking a car within the recreation area; there is a $7 daily fee to park here.) Parking Lot 11 is 1.6 miles down FM 2025, or 1.2 miles beyond the entrance to Double Lake Recreation Area.

To reach Big Creek Scenic Area and gravel **LSHT Trailhead Parking Lot 12** (near LSHT mile 79.9) from the town of Shepherd, along US 59, head west on TX 150 for about 5 miles. Forest Service (FS) Road 217 is a small, paved road that comes in from the left—turn left (southeast) on FS 217 and follow it 1.8 miles. Parking Lot 12 will be on your right. A short side trail leads to the LSHT from the parking lot. Nonpotable water can be found in Big Creek, just a short walk westbound on the LSHT.

To reach the eastern end of Section 9 (LSHT mile 82.5), at **LSHT Tarkington Trailhead Parking Lot 13**

A pretty creek surrounded by a variety of trees in Big Creek Scenic Area

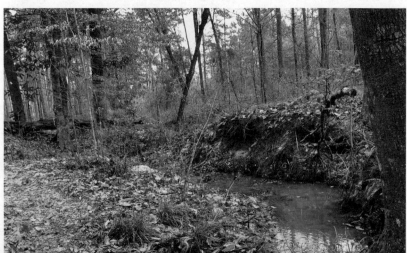

along FM 2666, from the town of Shepherd, along US 59, head west on TX 150 for about 1.5 miles. FM 2666 meets TX 150 on the left—turn left onto FM 2666, and follow it 6.5 miles. Parking Lot 13 is signed and visible on the right side of the road. There is ample parking, a trash can, and a bulletin board, but no drinking water.

SECTION 9 GPS Waypoints	
Double Lake Recreation Area, mile 75.0	N30° 32.759' W95° 07.833'
Primitive Campsite 1, mile 75.7	N30° 32.466' W95° 07.419'
LSHT Big Creek Trailhead Parking Lot 12, Big Creek Scenic Area	N30° 30.333' W95° 05.314'
LSHT Tarkington Trailhead Parking Lot 13, FM 2666	N30° 29.558' W95° 07.111'

SUPPLIES AND ACCOMMODATIONS

Double Lake Recreation Area has campsites (starting at $20 per night) equipped with picnic tables and campfire rings or a cooking grill. Hot showers, bathrooms with running water, and potable-water taps are located throughout the campground, as are vending machines. A concession stand operates during the warmer months on weekends. During this time of year, camping reservations are recommended (see Appendix A, page 155). These facilities are a few minutes' walk from the LSHT: from mile 75 and the large LSHT sign by the southwest corner of the lake, turn left and head into the campground, which is visible from this spot (the LSHT continues to the right).

The town of **Coldspring** (population 853), about 4 miles northeast of Double Lake on TX 150, has rental cottages, several restaurants, a post office, a dollar store, a couple of gas stations, and a large grocery store. The larger, full-service town of **Shepherd** (population: 2,319),

11 miles southeast of Coldspring along US 59, has similar amenities, along with several motels.

Shepherd can also be accessed from the eastern or southern end of LSHT Section 9. From FM 2666 and LSHT Trailhead Parking Lot 13, follow FM 2666 about 6.5 miles east. Turn right (east) on TX 150, and follow it 1.5 miles into Shepherd. Or, from LSHT Trailhead Parking Lot 12 in Big Creek Scenic Area, follow FS 217 northeast a few miles to the intersection with TX 150; Shepherd is about 5 miles to the east.

WATER

The Big Creek Section is blessed with abundant water. At the shoreline of spring-fed Double Lake, it's a short walk off-trail to its developed recreation facilities (including potable tap water) at the western end Section 9, at mile 75.

As you head into the middle part of this section, the trail parallels Double Lake Branch and, later, Big Creek. These spring-fed creeks flow year-round with clear water that is easily the most appealing of any groundwater along the entire LSHT. Good water becomes more scarce, however, toward the eastern end of Section 9, from mile 79.8 to mile 82.3.

TRAIL DESCRIPTION

The LSHT intersects Double Lake on the shoreline at the far southwest corner of the lake by a large LSHT sign at MILE MARKER 75. The LSHT skirts but does not enter Double Lake Recreation Area's facilities. The trail continues east from the large LSHT sign at mile 75—while facing the lake at the sign, make a hard right back into the woods to formally enter Section 9. *Do not continue straight ahead on the trail across the lake's dam.* (Remember that if you're hiking from east to west, you need to reverse all directions, left and right, in these trail descriptions.)

You soon cross a utilities right-of-way and intersect one of the recreation area's mountain biking trails. At mile 75.3, meet up with a short boardwalk over a wet section. Cross an old fenceline to reach another short boardwalk; notice a transition into picturesque moist woodland dominated by evergreen shrubs, vines, and ferns. Cross gravel FS 220 and proceed through a hiker gate across the road and over a large creek that drains Double Lake at mile 75.6—this is a main tributary of Big Creek named Double Lake Branch, which you follow for the next 4 miles (though mostly at a distance). Cross a tiny bridge over a seasonal drainage to reach designated LSHT Primitive Campsite 1 Ⓐ at mile 75.7, which has four tent pads. Damage to large trees in this area is probably due to past storms. If there are too many damaged trees to make camp here safe, don't worry; there are places to make a backcountry camp throughout the area just ahead. ▲ Water can usually be found by hiking downhill to Double Lake Branch. 🜄🜄🜄

Ⓐ **Campsite**

▲ **Campsite**
🜄 **Water**

The LSHT turns slightly uphill and then enters a higher, more open woodland of loblolly pine where camping is also possible. ▲ MILE MARKER 76 appears just after a precarious-looking hiker bridge over a steep-walled drainage. 🜊 Reach another deep drainage and another small hiker bridge again at mile 76.4. Soon cross yet another creek 🜊 whose bridge was washed out by the 2017 floods caused by Hurricane Harvey. Many of the bridges ahead in this section were in fact washed out by the tremendous flooding in 2017, but they've since been replaced or repaired. Without them, hikers would have a much more difficult time enjoying the picturesque woods and clear creeks in this area.

▲ **Campsite**

🜊 **Water**

If you have a sharp eye for trees, you may notice a pure stand of swamp chestnut oaks (*Quercus michauxii*). Mature leaves can be up to 11 inches long (though they're typically between 4 and 8 inches in length), broad, and oval, with rounded teeth. The large acorns of this bottomland-dwelling oak taste extra sweet to livestock, giving this tree its nickname of "cow oak." As you proceed along the banks of Double Lake Branch, ⚡ you also pass Southern magnolias, American hollies, red oaks, beeches, sycamores, and hickories, to name only a few of the tree species that thrive in this section.

Water ⚡

Pass a set of bridges just before **MILE MARKER 77**, located high and to the right in a big pine tree. Cross a small drainage and proceed along the side of the hill. Cross the creek again at mile 77.6, where the water tends to stagnate at times, making it an excellent area for wildflowers in the spring. Just 0.1 mile past **MILE MARKER 78**, a large, open area on the banks of Double Lake Branch makes a good place for a picnic; this pretty spot is below and to the left of the LSHT as it curves on a hillside above the creek. The LSHT was rerouted more than a decade ago from a lower course closer to the creek to higher ground, helping prevent damage to the trail and better protecting the creek's sensitive banks during seasonal flooding.

At mile 78.6 cross an old railroad trestle, following signs to the left. You are now entering Big Creek Scenic Area, where no campfire building, camping, or hunting is allowed—look for camping again after LSHT mile 80.6, but keep in mind that there's no other designated camping in this section during deer-hunting season. The trail can be very muddy through here, but hiker bridges and boardwalks cover the worst areas. Look for **MILE MARKER 79** just after a bridge near where a huge beech carved with thoughtless (but thankfully faded) graffiti grows to the right of the trail. Mosquitoes frequent this area even in cooler months.

Reach the junction of Double Lake Branch with Big Creek's other main tributary, Henry Lake Branch. A little waterfall graces this spot. A sign tells you that you've come

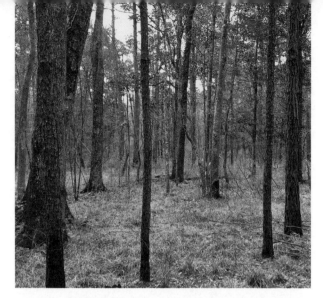

Set in a mixed pine–hardwood forest, Section 9 is the most ecologically diverse segment of the LSHT.

4 miles since Double Lake, which is fairly accurate. Cross a big bridge and intersect the orange-blazed Big Creek Trail, which heads off to the right. Next you'll see a signed junction with the green-blazed White Oak Trail, which also heads off to the right—stay straight on the LSHT, and immediately cross a bridge over Big Creek's clear waters. ◊◊◊◊◊ Pass ◊ **Water** a tiny bridge, and follow the LSHT to the right and through a muddy area where butterflies frolic among wildflowers in the spring. A long hiker bridge slopes slightly but is passable at mile 79.5. Continue to parallel spring-fed Big Creek, which is to the right. With beech trees leaning over its banks and clear, deep waters, Big Creek is especially scenic. Eastbound overnight hikers should consider treating water here if conditions are dry, as no reliable water is available for the next 13 miles.

Cross another long bridge and then reach a junction with the yellow-striped Pine Trail, which heads off to the right—follow the LSHT to the left. Cross another bridge and then, at LSHT mile 79.9, make a sharp right where you should see a large sign with a map of Big Creek Scenic Area on it. Another trail heads left to LSHT Big Creek Scenic

Area Trailhead Parking Lot 12, which has a bench and information board.

ALTERNATIVE BIG CREEK SCENIC AREA LOOP TRAILS

PINE TRAIL Yellow-blazed, 0.1-mile one-way, 0.75-mile loop

WHITE OAK TRAIL Green-blazed, 0.4-mile one-way, 1.5-mile loop

BIG CREEK TRAIL Orange-blazed, 0.6-mile one-way, 2-mile loop

Past the junction noted on the previous page, the trail begins a southwestern arc; eastbound hikers may notice that they're heading due west for a few miles before turning south. As you continue on the LSHT, you may notice a yellow-blazed trail, the other end of the Pine Trail, heading off to the right, followed by a couple of trailside benches and the orange-striped Big Creek Trail off to the right. (The White Oak Trail also joins the LSHT again at this point.)

Soon, reach **MILE MARKER 80**. If you haven't already noticed, you're walking on top of an old rail bed that once served the logging industry. Pass a peaceful bench at 80.6; then proceed straight across gravel FS 221 at mile 80.9, leaving Big Creek Scenic Area. Immediately, Big Creek's diverse ecosystem is replaced by a homogenous young pine plantation.

Pass **MILE MARKER 81**, where a large, open area to the left could make a waterless camp, ▲ and then cross a small seasonal drainage. At mile 81.2, follow the LSHT left; you could also make a waterless camp ▲ in another open spot here. Cross several more seasonal drainages in hardwood bottomland, including the unbridged, ephemeral upper channel of Tarkington Bayou ⏚ at mile 81.5. A nearby old

Campsite ▲

Campsite ▲

Water ⏚

oxbow of the bayou could be used as an in-a-pinch water source for very thirsty hikers who find Tarkington dry.

Continue to walk in and out of hardwood bottomland and young pine forests. At mile 81.9, look for another small, waterless campsite ▲ just before you enter a mature forest of white ash, black hickory, and white oak. Then reach **MILE MARKER 82** and continue on to LSHT Trailhead Parking Lot 13, along FM 2666 at LSHT mile 82.5.

▲ Campsite

MILES W→E	TRAIL POINT	MILES E→W	NOTES
75.0	Double Lake Recreation Area; **MILE MARKER 75**	21.4	⛲🚻 Ⓐ 🅿
75.1	Utilities right-of-way; intersect mountain bike trail	21.3	
75.6	Gravel FS 220; hiker gate; Double Lake Branch on left (good water, medium flow 💧💧💧)	20.8	⛲ 💧
75.7	Hiker bridge over seasonal drainage; LSHT Primitive Campsite 1	20.7	Ⓐ
76.0	Bridge over deep drainage; potential camping; seasonal creek on left (good water, low flow 🚰); **MILE MARKER 76**	20.4	🚰 ▲
76.4	Small bridge over deep drainage	20.0	
76.6	Ford wide seasonal creek (bridge destroyed in 2017; low flow, good water 🚰)	19.8	🚰
76.9	Two bridges over seasonal creeks (low flow, good water 🚰)	19.5	🚰
77.0	**MILE MARKER 77**	19.4	
77.6	Cross swampy creek (stagnant water)	18.8	
78.0	**MILE MARKER 78**	18.4	
78.1	Picnic spot off LSHT along banks of Double Lake Branch	18.3	
78.6	Cross old rail bed; left on LSHT	17.8	
79.0	**MILE MARKER 79**	17.4	
79.2	Intersect orange-blazed Big Creek Trail; left on LSHT	17.2	
79.3	Intersect green-blazed White Oak Trail; left on LSHT	17.1	
79.4	Bridge over Big Creek (high flow, good water 💧💧💧💧💧)	17.0	💧
79.7	Long bridge over Big Creek; intersect yellow-blazed Pine Trail; left on LSHT	16.7	💧

continued on next page

SECTION 9 Mileage

MILES W→E	TRAIL POINT	MILES E→W	NOTES
79.8	Hiker bridge; intersect trail heading down to left; sharp right on LSHT	16.6	
79.9	BIG CREEK SCENIC AREA sign; short side trail to left leads to LSHT Trailhead Parking Lot 12; intersect yellow-blazed Pine Trail and orange-blazed Big Creek Trail on right; straight on LSHT on old rail bed	16.5	🅿
80.0	**MILE MARKER 80**	16.4	
80.6	Bench; potential waterless camp	15.8	▲
80.9	FS 221	15.5	⚬⚬
81.0	**MILE MARKER 81**; potential waterless camp	15.4	▲
81.2	Intersect unidentified trail; left on LSHT; potential campsite; seasonal drainage	15.2	▲
81.5	Upper reaches of Tarkington Bayou (seasonal flow, good water 🚰)	14.9	🚰
82.0	**MILE MARKER 82**	14.4	
82.5	LSHT Tarkington Trailhead Parking Lot 13; FM 2666	13.9	⚬⚬ 🅿

MILEAGE CHART KEY

▲	Undeveloped campsite or potential camping area	🚰	Water source (seasonal/unrated)
Ⓐ	Designated campsite during hunting season	⚬⚬	Major roads (jeep tracks and logging roads not indicated)
◊	Water source (DROPS-rated)	🅿	Parking area/trailhead

FM 2666 TO FM 1725

OVERVIEW

THE WORD *BAYOU* probably originated from the Choctaw word for "small stream" and was first used by the French in the Louisiana Territory to denote a slow-moving creek in a relatively flat, low area. Section 10 provides hikers with the opportunity for an up-close encounter with a small East Texas bayou named Tarkington and its rich ecosystem.

Popular culture has often cast bayous in the role of spooky, mysterious places where overhanging moss darkens foreboding, junglelike forests. Come out and hike this section of the LSHT to see for yourself—you'll find, as you stroll along the banks of Tarkington Bayou, that bayous and their surrounding lands are unique. Indeed, many forest creatures depend on their slow-moving waters for homes. Trees of all types live in these bottomlands, and plants uncommon in other sections of the LSHT—leafy vines, ferns, and palms—are abundant here. Be cognizant of recent weather conditions, though, as these lowlands tend to fill with standing, sometimes flowing water when rains drench the area.

TRAIL ACCESS AND PARKING

The two parking lots in Section 10 have ample parking and an information board, but they lack drinking water and trash collection.

LSHT Tarkington Trailhead Parking Lot 13 is located at the western (or northern) end of Section 10 (at LSHT mile 82.5). To reach it, head west from the town of Shepherd along TX 150. About 1.5 miles after leaving the intersection of US 59 and TX 150, turn left on FM 2666

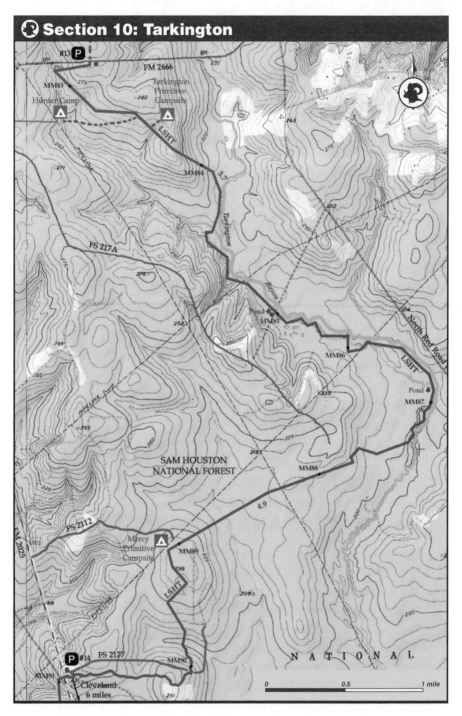

and follow it for 6.5 miles. The signed parking lot is on the right side of FM 2666.

To reach **LSHT Trailhead Parking Lot 14,** also called the **Mercy Fire Tower Trailhead,** take FM 2025 about 7 miles northwest from the town of Cleveland. The parking lot is on the right side of FM 2025 at LSHT mile 90.9.

SECTION 10 GPS Waypoints	
LSHT Tarkington Trailhead Parking Lot 13, FM 2666	N30° 29.558' W95° 07.111'
LSHT Mercy Fire Tower Trailhead Parking Lot 14, FM 2025	N30° 26.312' W95° 07.268'

SUPPLIES AND ACCOMMODATIONS

The full-service town of **Shepherd** (population 2,319), about 8 miles from the eastern end of Section 9, has motels, restaurants, a post office, and many other amenities. From FM 2666 and LSHT Trailhead Parking Lot 13, follow FM 2666 about 6.5 miles east. Turn right (east) on TX 150, and follow it 1.5 miles into Shepherd.

The larger town of **Cleveland** (population 7,954), about 6 miles southeast of LSHT Trailhead Parking Lot 14 at the junction of FM 2025 and US 59, also has several motels along with a good selection of stores and restaurants.

A well-equipped gas station and convenience store (which sells sandwiches and minor medical supplies), as well as a **Dollar General** store, are close to the trail. The gas station is 0.9 mile south-southeast of Parking Lot 14 on FM 2025, and Dollar General is 2.7 miles south-southeast of Parking Lot 14 on FM 2025.

WATER

Tarkington Bayou, which the LSHT follows for approximately 3 miles, is intermittent and cannot be relied upon in any season. A pond and oxbow at miles 85 and 86.4 are more reliable, though perhaps not as enticing.

TRAIL DESCRIPTION

From LSHT Trailhead Parking Lot 13, along FM 2666 at LSHT mile 82.3, cross the highway and continue to parallel it on the trail for a few minutes in piney woods. The rolling land you've experienced since crossing the East Fork of the San Jacinto River back in Section 8 (if you're thru-hiking) is now gone—instead, you walk through long stretches of pure pine forests on flat ground. Longleaf pines, rare along the LSHT, grow in this area. These trees are highly resistant to fire and, before the suppression of wildfires by European settlers, were the dominant pines in the southern US. Today, longleaf pines grow in only 5% of their former range.

Pass **MILE MARKER 83** among brushy undergrowth. At mile 83.5, you may notice a corner benchmark near a side trail to the right that leads to a designated (approved for **Campsite ⏃** use during deer season) camp in 0.6 mile. ⏃ A few minutes later, reach primitive Tarkington Campsite, ⏃ another designated site 100 yards to the left of the trail (*note:* no water available). Cross a seasonal drainage on a hiker bridge at mile 83.7, followed by another drainage without a bridge close to **MILE MARKER 84**. The trail drops gradually as it heads toward the bottomlands of Tarkington Bayou.

Water ⧫ At mile 84.3 reach Tarkington Bayou, ⧫ which at first looks like any other small seasonal creek but is often bone-dry in warm, dry weather. Here, you're within 5 miles of its headwaters. As you continue, you cross a hiker bridge **Water ⛲** at mile 84.6 over a seasonal tributary. ⛲ You could set up a small campsite on the right side of the trail at mile **Campsite ▲** 84.9. ▲ Near mile 85, the dam of a small pond ⧫⧫⧫ **Water ⧫** should be visible from the trail 50 yards to the east (left) of the LSHT. Right after you pass **MILE MARKER 85**, cross a pipeline and its access road to enter mature woodland. The trail meanders alongside the bayou, which remains on your left, and eventually passes **MILE MARKER 86**. (Remember that if you're hiking westbound, you need to reverse all directions, left and right, in these trail descriptions.)

At mile 86.1 cross a small ditch that can overflow after heavy rains. Two signs mark a left turn at 86.2 and then a sharp right turn at 86.3. In some years the bayou's waters may recede underground for a while, leaving hikers without a water supply, save for some old murky oxbows, like the one at mile 86.4. ⬡⬡⬡ You might notice a very tall magnolia tree to the left a few minutes before you pass

⬡ **Water**

This majestic magnolia stands at mile 86.4.

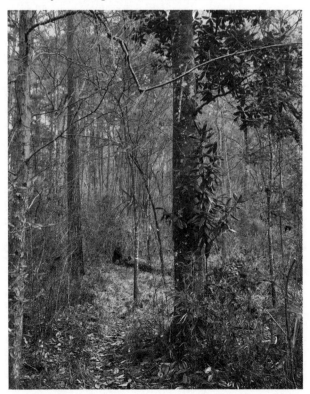

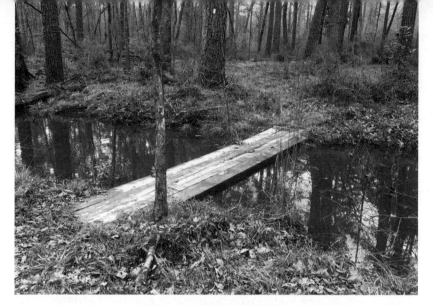

A rough-hewn hiker bridge crosses Tarkington Bayou at mile 87.1.

MILE MARKER 87. Cross a crude hiker bridge at mile 87.1. Even if the bayou is dry here, it continues to be an easy, picturesque walk through a mature pine-dominated forest. Veer away from the bayou for good, having never crossed it, by mile 87.6.

Pass **MILE MARKER 88** and then cross a pipeline right-of-way at 88.3 on a straight path through a young pine forest. Cross a seasonal drainage at mile 88.7. Not far after passing **MILE MARKER 89**, turn left onto a logging road. Signs here lead to designated Mercy Primitive **Campsite ⚠** Campsite, ⚠ 100 feet to the right of the trail and adjacent to FS 2112, which is closed to traffic. A fire ring, dry tent sites, and a wooden bench make this a great camping option, especially in wet weather.

Watch for a sharp right turn at mile 89.3; the trail still appears to follow the logging road. The forest has grown more mature with thick scrub brush as undergrowth. You may be able to spot more longleaf pines in this area. Cross a hiker bridge at a seasonal wetland and creek where a farmstead is visible off to the left. Just past **MILE MARKER 90**, the trail crosses crudely paved Forest Valley Drive near private property. Dogs may bark at you here.

Cross a series of abandoned jeep tracks, one of which you follow. At least one of these junctions can be confusing if you're hiking eastbound as there are few trail markers: at the junction, veer slightly to the right, but don't take a hard right; then keep straight. At mile 90.2, in a mix of trees including hollies and magnolias, look for a small clearing with space for one waterless campsite. ▲

▲ **Campsite**

Reach FM 2025, which runs north–south, at mile 90.9. (The LSHT here has turned westward briefly.) LSHT Trailhead Parking Lot 14 is located along FM 2025. Thru-hikers may be interested to know that the gas station with the convenience store is located 0.9 mile to the left (south–southeast), at the junction of FM 2025 and FM 945; the Dollar General store is 2.7 miles in the same direction from the parking lot.

SECTION 10 Mileage

MILES W→E	TRAIL POINT	MILES E→W	NOTES
82.5	LSHT Trailhead Parking Lot 13; FM 2666	13.9	➖ 🅿
83.0	**MILE MARKER 83**	13.4	
83.5	Corner benchmark and bearing tree; 0.6-mi side trail to designated campsite	12.9	Ⓐ
83.6	Designated campsite	12.8	Ⓐ
83.7	Bridge over creek (stagnant water)	12.7	
84.0	**MILE MARKER 84**; seasonal drainage	12.4	
84.3	Reach banks of Tarkington Bayou ⬣	12.1	⬣
84.6	Hiker bridge over seasonal creek 🚰	11.8	🚰
84.9	Potential campsite	11.5	▲
85.0	**MILE MARKER 85**; pond ⬣⬣⬣ 50 yd east; pipeline and access road	11.4	⬣
86.0	**MILE MARKER 86**	10.4	
86.2	Old logging road; follow LSHT left, then right	10.2	
86.4	Oxbow pond of Tarkington Bayou (muddy) ⬣⬣⬣	10.0	⬣

continued on next page

SECTION 10 Mileage

MILES W→E	TRAIL POINT	MILES E→W	NOTES
87.0	**MILE MARKER 87**	9.4	
87.6	Veer away from Tarkington Bayou for good	8.8	
88.0	**MILE MARKER 88**	8.4	
88.3	Pipeline right-of-way	8.1	
88.7	Seasonal drainage	7.7	
89.0	**MILE MARKER 89;** left on logging road; Mercy Primitive Campsite	7.4	ⓐ
89.3	Sharp turn to right	7.1	
90.0	**MILE MARKER 90;** semipaved Forest Valley Dr. near private homes	6.4	▬
90.1	Abandoned jeep roads; confusing junction; follow LSHT slightly to right and then straight	6.3	
90.2	Potential waterless campsite	6.2	▲
90.9	FM 2025; LSHT Trailhead Parking Lot 14 (store 0.9 mi south)	5.5	▬ 🅿

MILEAGE CHART KEY

▲	Undeveloped campsite or potential camping area	🚰	Water source (seasonal/unrated)
ⓐ	Designated campsite during hunting season	▬▬▬	Major roads (jeep tracks and logging roads not indicated)
💧	Water source (DROPS-rated)	🅿	Parking area/trailhead

FARM TO MARKET 2666 TO FARM TO MARKET 1725

OVERVIEW

THE WINTERS BAYOU SECTION traverses the lowest elevation along the entire LSHT—about 160 feet above sea level—so not only is the trail blessed with many creeks and drainages, but it also tends to flood during wet seasons. After heavy rains, in fact, expect to be wading in ankle-deep water in some places. This section's two large waterways are bridged with dependable steel-foot bridges, but after large amounts of rainfall, hikers should be aware that these small rivers can sweep over their banks. This section is best enjoyed during drier times.

Hikers will encounter a primeval landscape of beautiful lowlands that harbor a wide variety of trees and wildflowers in season, including orchids. Winters Bayou, which drains a large portion of Sam Houston National Forest, is recognized as an ecologically significant stream. With very little pastureland or development in its drainage and several spring-fed tributaries, the bayou's high water quality and rich landscape provide prime habitats to a diverse range of aquatic life. For these reasons, the area is protected as a special scenic area within the national forest.

Unfortunately, there are no designated (approved) campsites along the LSHT in this short section, making it impossible to legally camp along the trail here during deer-hunting season from late September through early January.

TRAIL ACCESS AND PARKING

To reach **LSHT Trailhead Parking Lot 14,** also called the **Mercy Fire Tower Trailhead,** take FM 2025 approximately 7 miles northwest from Cleveland. The parking lot is on the right side of the road at LSHT mile 90.9.

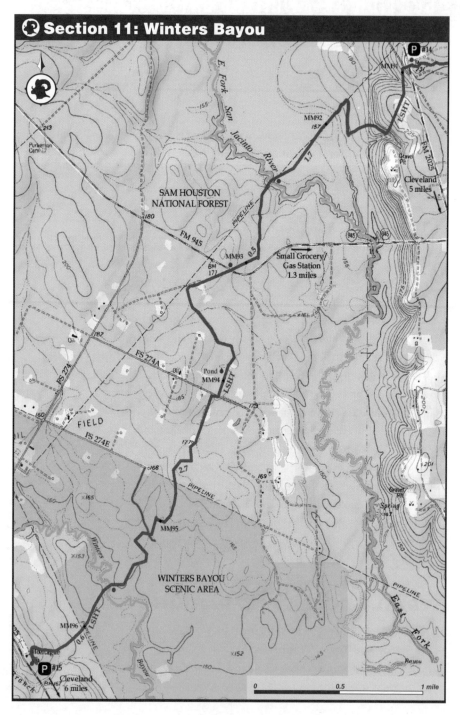

To reach the LSHT crossing of TX 945 (at LSHT mile 93.1) from Cleveland along US 59, follow FM 2025 north for 6.5 miles to the junction with TX 945 (look for a gas station on the left at this intersection). Turn onto TX 945 and go 1.4 miles, watching for LSHT signs pointing out the location of the trail as it crosses the road. There is neither a parking lot nor a trailhead here.

To reach the eastern, or southern, end and terminus of the LSHT (at mile 96.1) on FM 1725 from Cleveland, follow TX 105 for 1 mile west from US 59. Turn right (northwest) onto FM 1725, and go 5.2 miles to reach **LSHT Trailhead Parking Lot 15,** also known as the **Winters Bayou Trailhead,** on the right side of the road just before a white church building (Montague Church).

SECTION 11 GPS Waypoints	
LSHT Mercy Fire Tower Trailhead Parking Lot 14, FM 2025	N30° 26.312' W95° 07.268'
LSHT crossing of San Jacinto River on steel hiker bridge, mile 92.6	N30° 25.771' W95° 08.100'
Intersection with TX 945, mile 93.1	N30° 25.381' W95° 08.328'
LSHT Winters Bayou Trailhead Parking Lot 15, FM 1725	N30° 23.593' W95° 09.484'

SUPPLIES AND ACCOMMODATIONS

The full-service town of **Cleveland** (population 7,954), about 6 miles southeast of LSHT Trailhead Parking Lot 14 at the junction of FM 2025 and US 59, has several motels and a good selection of stores and restaurants. Cleveland can also be reached easily from the LSHT crossing of TX 945 (LSHT mile 93.1) by heading east on TX 945 for 1.4 miles and then heading south on FM 2025 for 6.5 miles.

From the eastern terminus of the LSHT (mile 96.4) and LSHT Trailhead Parking Lot 15, you can reach Cleveland by taking FM 1725 southeast for 5.2 miles and then heading east on TX 105 for 1 mile. When you reach US Highway 59, turn north and drive about 1 mile to reach the town center.

A well-stocked gas station and convenience store (which sells sandwiches and minor medical supplies), as well as a **Dollar General** store, are close to the trail. The gas station is 0.9 mile south-southeast of Parking Lot 14 on FM 2025 and 1.3 miles east of the LSHT crossing on FM 945; Dollar General is 2.7 miles south-southeast of Parking Lot 14 along FM 2025.

WATER

Section 11's large, reliable water sources can be intimidating to reach and treat. The perennial East Fork of the San Jacinto River and Winters Bayou both hold muddy water and have steep, slippery banks. A small creek and pond at mile 93.8 contain water in all but the driest conditions. Several smaller tributaries and streams feed into these bottomlands, many of which flow clear and strong most of the year but cannot be relied upon in very dry seasons.

TRAIL DESCRIPTION

The Winters Bayou section begins where LSHT enters the woods directly across from Parking Lot 14 on FM 2025. You reach **MILE MARKER 91** within a few minutes. After crossing a seasonal drainage, enter a hardwood forest dominated by white oak and hickory. A few open areas under pines present themselves as potential waterless campsites. ▲

Campsite ▲

Parallel a seasonal drainage, and then cross a small creek that may harbor water 🚰 at mile 91.4. You're about to head downhill into the bottomlands of the East Fork of the San Jacinto—your second crossing of the river if you're thru-hiking eastbound. At around mile 91.6, turn

Water 🚰

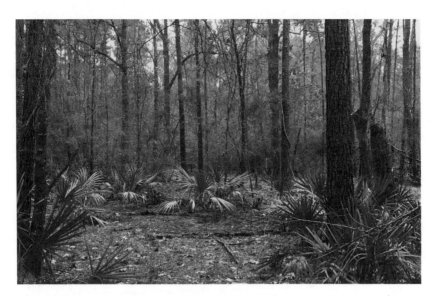

Palmetto bottomlands near FM 945

right and follow an old rail bed for a few hundred feet. In the next 0.5 mile, you pass many water oaks and swamp chestnut oaks, both water-tolerant species.

Reach a small seasonal creek 🚰 that might have good water in it just before **MILE MARKER 92**. Note that you may have to hop over this creek, or cross on a downed log if it's running hard. The palmetto bottomlands through here flood regularly, so be prepared to wade through ankle-deep water if the season has been wet.

Just after you cross another seasonal creek, you should spot the muddy waters of the East Fork of the San Jacinto River on the right. ⬡⬡⬡⬡⬡ Reach the large steel hiker bridge spanning the river at mile 92.6. You could set up potential campsites on the opposite bank, ▲ but it would be difficult and potentially dangerous to scramble down to the river here to get water—be very cautious and consider other water sources instead. Follow a dirt road straight ahead, watching for the trail to head off into the woods to the left within 0.1 mile.

🚰 **Water**

⬡ **Water**

▲ **Campsite**

Pass through a wetland area where buttonbush (a shrub with greenish white flowers) and blue waterleaf (a deep blue flower with five petals) bloom in the spring. In a young pine forest, cross an often stagnant creek at mile 92.7. The trail is open and pleasant in this area, but you can expect some large standing puddles in wet seasons. At **MILE MARKER 93**, cross a small hiker bridge over a wetland. Soon afterward, reach TX 945 and cross it on a diagonal to the right. There is no official trail parking here; however, thru-hikers may be interested to know that there is a combination gas station/convenience store 1.3 miles away at the intersection of TX 945 and FM 2025, as well as a Dollar General 1.7 miles south-southeast on FM 2025 from the gas station. Eastbounders will turn left (east) on FM 945 to reach the gas station.

Water ◊

Water ⌑

At mile 93.4 you may notice the concrete pillars of an old lookout tower's base. At mile 93.8 look for a small creek and pond ◊◊◊ to the right (north) of the trail. You may later be distracted and not notice **MILE MARKER 94** by another fire-tower base adjacent to a creek ⌑ that may have clear, running water in it. Take a sharp right on an old road (FS 274B), walk a little ways down it, and then take a hard left—the road continues straight ahead, so be careful not to stay on it. The trail may be wet in this area even though it now follows another older roadbed. Pass yet another fire-tower base at mile 94.5.

Cross well-maintained gravel FS 274A at mile 94.7. These forests are comprised of mostly hardwoods; the wet soil also lends itself to the growth of ferns, vines, and dwarf palmettos. Hikers who have a good eye may spot the elusive Louisiana palm (*Sabal louisiana*), which is uncommon in Texas. Often confused with the dwarf palmetto when young, the Louisiana palm can grow as tall as 18 feet (though it's usually 3–6 feet tall), with a trunk 2 feet in diameter. (The common dwarf palmetto is also considered a palm but does not have a trunk.)

A few minutes after you pass **MILE MARKER 95**, cross a gravel road, followed by a hiker bridge over a seasonal creek. Sadly, this road leads to an oil-and-gas well drilled in the heart of Winters Bayou Scenic Area. At mile 95.2, a long boardwalk damaged by Hurricane Harvey's flooding in late 2017 takes you through a palmetto swamp. Farther on, another bridge helps keep your feet dry over a wetland. These are the bottomlands of Winters Bayou, another large creek that joins the East Fork of the San Jacinto about 3 miles downstream from here.

Reach the banks of Winters Bayou (◊◊◊◊◊   ◊ **Water** elevation 135'), and cross it on another large steel bridge at mile 95.8. Then, at mile 95.9, cross a shallow oxbow on a bridge that was also flood-damaged in 2017. In a few hundred feet, you'll walk under overhead phone lines, pass **MILE MARKER 96**, and cross over another bridged wetland. One final bridge leads over a wet area at mile 96.1. Now the trail takes you under the boughs of young trees before meeting up with older forest. Very large Southern magnolias and white oaks grow here.

Once you spot the white church and barbwire fence, you're at mile 96.4. LSHT Trailhead Parking Lot 15, a large gravel area off FM 1725, is the eastern terminus of the Lone Star Hiking Trail. Congratulations, eastbound thru-hikers!

SECTION 11 Mileage

MILES W→E	TRAIL POINT	MILES E→W	NOTES
90.9	FM 2025; LSHT Trailhead Parking Lot 14 (store 1 mi south)	5.5	▭ 🅿
91.0	**MILE MARKER 91**	5.4	
91.2	Potential camping	5.2	▲
91.4	Cross at junction of small creeks (low flow, clear water, unreliable 🚰)	5.0	🚰
91.6	Right on old rail bed	4.8	

continued on next page

SECTION 11 Mileage

MILES W→E	TRAIL POINT	MILES E→W	NOTES
92.0	Unbridged seasonal creek (clear water 🚰); **MILE MARKER 92**	4.4	🚰
92.6	Steel hiker bridge over East Fork of the San Jacinto River (deep, muddy water) 💧💧💧💧💧	3.8	💧
92.7	Seasonal creek (stagnant water)	3.7	
93.0	**MILE MARKER 93**; bridge over wetland	3.4	
93.1	TX 945 (store 1.3 mi east)	3.3	▬
93.4	Old fire-tower base	3.0	
93.8	Creek; 💧 small pond on right (north)	2.6	💧
94.0	Creek (clear water, seasonal flow 🚰); **MILE MARKER 94**; old fire-tower base	2.4	🚰
94.5	Old fire-tower base	1.9	
94.7	Gravel FS 274A	1.7	
95.0	**MILE MARKER 95**; pipeline with road; hiker bridge over seasonal creek	1.4	
95.2	Boardwalk over palmetto swamp	1.2	
95.8	Steel hiker bridge over Winters Bayou (deep, muddy water) 💧💧💧💧💧	0.6	💧
95.9	Phone lines; boardwalk over wet area	0.5	
96.0	**MILE MARKER 96**	0.4	
96.1	Bridge over shallow drainage	0.3	
96.4	LSHT Trailhead Parking Lot 15; FM 1725; eastern terminus of LSHT	0.0	▬ 🅿

MILEAGE CHART KEY

▲	Undeveloped campsite or potential camping area	🚰	Water source (seasonal/unrated)
Ⓐ	Designated campsite during hunting season	▬▬▬	Major roads (jeep tracks and logging roads not indicated)
💧	Water source (DROPS-rated)	🅿	Parking area/trailhead

APPENDIXES

<hr>

APPENDIX A: RESOURCES AND CONTACT INFORMATION

Lone Star Hiking Trail Club, Inc.
lonestartrail.org
113 Ben Drive
Houston, TX 77022

Double Lake Recreation Area
tinyurl.com/doublelake
301 FM 2025
Coldspring, TX 77331
936-653-3448
Camping reservations: 877-444-6777,
recreation.gov/camping/campgrounds/232430

Huntsville State Park
tpwd.texas.gov/state-parks/huntsville
565 Park Road 40 W.
Huntsville, TX 77340
936-295-5644

National Forest Maps
NATIONAL FORESTS AND GRASSLANDS IN TEXAS
tinyurl.com/nfgtmaps

Sam Houston National Forest
tinyurl.com/samhoustonnationalforest
394 FM 1375 W.
New Waverly, TX 77358
936-344-6205, 888-361-6908
Office hours: Monday–Friday, 8 a.m.–4:30 p.m.

Sierra Club Houston Group
sierraclub.org/texas/houston
PO Box 3021
Houston, TX 77253-3021

Taxi Services
CLEVELAND
350 Cab 936-328-8181

CONROE
CVS Taxi Cab 936-537-5829
On Time Cab 936-539-1057

USGS Maps
store.usgs.gov/maps

EMERGENCY CONTACTS	
24-Hour Emergencies	911
Cleveland Regional Medical Center	281-593-1811
HCA Houston Healthcare Conroe	936-539-1111
Huntsville Memorial Hospital	936-291-3411
Huntsville Police Department	936-435-8001
Liberty County Sheriff's Office	281-592-3411
Montgomery County Sheriff's Office	936-760-5800
Sam Houston National Forest Law Enforcement Officer	936-827-5189 (cell), 936-639-7539 (office)
Sam Houston Ranger District	936-344-6205
San Jacinto County Sheriff's Office	936-653-4367
Walker County Sheriff's Office	936-435-8001

APPENDIX B: REFERENCES AND RECOMMENDED READING

Ajilvsgi, Geyata. *Wildflowers of Texas.* Fredericksburg, TX: Shearer Publishing, 1984.

American Association of University Women, North Harris County Branch. *The Heritage of North Harris County.* Houston: American Association of University Women, North Harris County Branch, 1977.

Cabeza de Vaca, Álvar Núñez. *Adventures in the Unknown Interior of America.* Translated by Cyclone Covey. Scotts Valley, CA: Amazon/CreateSpace, 2016.

Fletcher, Colin, and Chip Rawlins. *The Complete Walker IV.* New York City: Knopf, 2002.

Rappole, John H., and Gene W. Blacklock. *Birds of Texas.* Houston: Rice University Press, 1990.

Robison, B. C. *Birds of Houston.* Houston: Rice University Press, 1990.

Schimelpfenig, Todd, Linda Lindsey, and Joan Safford. *NOLS Wilderness First Aid.* Mechanicsburg, PA: Stackpole Books, 2000.

Truett, Joe C., and Daniel W. Lay. *Land of Bears and Honey: A Natural History of East Texas.* Austin: University of Texas Press, 1994.

Tull, Delena, and George Oxford Miller. *Lone Star Field Guide to Wildflowers, Trees, and Shrubs of Texas.* Houston: Gulf Publishing Company, 1991.

Tveten, John, and Gloria Tveten. *Wildflowers of Houston and Southeast Texas.* Austin: University of Texas Press, 1993.

Vines, Robert A. *Trees of East Texas.* Austin: University of Texas Press, 1977.

Watson, Geraldine Ellis. *Big Thicket Plant Ecology.* Denton: University of North Texas Press, 2006.

APPENDIX C: EQUIPMENT AND FOOD CHECKLISTS

Day-Hiking Equipment Checklist

BASICS	CLOTHING	FIRST AID	OPTIONAL
Backpack	Boots or hiking shoes	Adhesive "vet wrap"	Bandanna
Backpack rain cover	Fleece jacket	Adhesive bandages	Camera
Compass	Gloves	Antibiotic ointment	Cell phone
Guidebook and maps	Insoles	Blister treatment	Extra batteries
Headlamp or flashlight	Pants	Gauze	Eyeglasses or contact lenses
Insect repellent	Rain jacket	Lip balm	Fishing gear
Lighter or matches	Shorts	Pain reliever	Gaiters
Money and ID	Socks	Sunscreen	GPS unit
Pocketknife	Sun hat	Waterproof medical tape	Hiking poles
Sunscreen	T-shirt		Insect head net
Toilet paper	Warm hat or balaclava		Sock liners
Water containers			Sunglasses
Water filter or chemical treatment			Watch
Zip-top bags			

Backpacking Equipment Checklist

Note: Add these items to the day-hiking checklist above.

BASICS	CLOTHING	TOILETRIES	OPTIONAL
30 feet of cord or rope	Camp shoes (e.g., sandals)	Brush or comb	Earplugs
Cooking pot with lid	Extra pants	Dental floss	Extra zip-top bags
Duct tape	Extra shorts	Feminine-hygiene products	Insulated mug

BASICS	CLOTHING	TOILETRIES	OPTIONAL
Fuel	Extra socks	Hair tie or clip	Pack towel
Sleeping bag	Extra T-shirt	Hand sanitizer	Paper and pen
Sleeping pad	Extra underwear	Regular prescription medications	Phone charger
Spoon	Long underwear	Toothbrush and toothpaste	Plastic camp mirror
Stove			Solar charger
Tent/hammock/tarp (plus rain fly, tent poles, ground cloth, insect net, straps, and/or stakes)			Stuff sacks (for food, clothes, etc.)

Hiking and Backpacking Meal-Planning Ideas

BREAKFAST	LUNCH	SNACKS	DINNER
Bagels	Beef jerky	Candy or chocolate bars	Capellini pasta (with pesto)
Cereal, granola, or muesli	Bread products (e.g., tortillas, bagels, or pita)	Chips	Couscous
Dehydrated milk; instant coffee	Cheese	Dried or fresh fruit	Dried textured vegetable protein
Dried or fresh fruit	Dried seaweed	Energy bars	Freeze-dried backpacker meal
Freeze-dried backpacker meal	Hazelnut spread (Nutella)	Hot cocoa, tea, or powdered drink mixes	Fresh or dehydrated vegetables
Granola bars or energy bars	Peanut or almond butter	Nuts	Instant rice
Oatmeal	Small condiment packets (soy or hot sauce, ketchup, mayonnaise)	Pretzels	Instant soups
Peanut butter sandwich	Tuna or chicken in a pouch	Trail mix	Prepackaged rice or noodle meals
Powdered protein shakes	Whole-grain crackers or cookies		Spices and seasonings; olive oil (in a small plastic bottle)

APPENDIX D:
CONSOLIDATED MILEAGE OF THE LSHT

See the Mileage Chart Key (page 173) for a guide to the icons used in this table.

MILES W→E	TRAIL POINT	MILES E→W	NOTES
★ **SECTION 1**			
0.0·	Western terminus of LSHT, FS 219 at FM 149, LSHT Richards Trailhead Parking Lot 1	96.4	▬ 🅿
0.1	Little Lake Creek Loop Trail (orange-blazed) branches right; left on LSHT	96.3	
0.2	Utilities right-of-way	96.2	
0.3	Small pond (semiclear water ◊◊◊)	96.1	◊
0.4	Seasonal drainage on left	96.0	
1.0	**MILE MARKER 1**; potential camping	95.4	▲
1.3	Large seasonal drainage	95.1	
1.8	FS 203 (good dirt road)	94.6	▬
2.0	Small seasonal drainage; **MILE MARKER 2**	94.4	
2.1	Left on LSHT, parallel to FS 203	94.3	▬
2.2	Abandoned jeep road	94.2	
2.5	Small pond (semiclear water ◊◊◊◊◊); potential camping	93.9	◊ ▲
2.7	Large seasonal drainage	93.7	
3.0	**MILE MARKER 3**	93.4	
3.3	Junction with West Fork Trail (purple-blazed); large seasonal drainage	93.1	
3.4	FS 211 (good gravel road); LSHT Sandy Branch Trailhead Parking Lot 2; enter Little Lake Creek (LLC) Wilderness	93.0	▬ 🅿
3.5	Potential camping	92.9	▲
3.8	Wilderness Trail branches left (red-blazed); straight on LSHT	92.6	
4.0	**MILE MARKER 4**; creek (low volume; good water ◊◊◊◊)	92.4	◊
4.5	Large seasonal drainage (stagnant water)	91.9	
4.7	Potential camping	91.7	▲
5.0	**MILE MARKER 5**	91.4	
5.1	Intersect Sand Branch Trail (yellow-blazed; 0.5 mi+ to primitive camping and pond); left on LSHT	91.3	Ⓐ

MILES W→E	TRAIL POINT	MILES E→W	NOTES
5.9	Boardwalks over Little Lake Creek bottomland ⬦	90.5	⬦
6.0	**MILE MARKER 6**	90.4	
6.4	LLC Wilderness boundary; FS 231 (0.2 mi to designated camping)	90.0	▬ Ⓐ
6.7	Pole Creek Trail (blue-blazed) heads right; left on LSHT	89.7	
7.0	**MILE MARKER 7**	89.4	
7.2	Creek adjacent to trail (low volume, good water 🚰)	89.2	🚰
7.7	Hiker bridge over deep drainage	88.7	
8.0	**MILE MARKER 8;** Pole Creek (low volume, good water 🚰); junction with North Wilderness Trail	88.4	▬ 🚰
8.6	Utilities right-of-way	87.8	
8.7	FM 149, LSHT North Wilderness Trailhead Parking Lot 3	87.7	▬ 🅿
★ **SECTION 2**			
8.7	FM 149, LSHT North Wilderness Trailhead Parking Lot 3	87.7	▬ 🅿
8.9	Junction of trails; left on LSHT	87.5	
9.0	**MILE MARKER 9**	87.4	
9.1	Jeep track; left on LSHT	87.3	
9.3	Junction of trails; left on LSHT; potential camping	87.1	▲
9.8	Pond (hard to see) on left ⬦⬦⬦⬦	86.6	⬦
10.0	**MILE MARKER 10**	86.4	
10.5	Potential waterless campsites	85.9	▲
10.9	T-junction; right on LSHT	85.5	
11.0	**MILE MARKER 11**	85.4	
11.3	FS 237/Osborn Rd.; trailhead parking	85.1	▬ 🅿
11.4	Utilities right-of-way	85.0	
11.8	Little Lake Creek Loop (orange-blazed) branches right; designated camping in 0.5 mi	84.6	Ⓐ
11.9	Caney Creek (high volume, good water ⬦⬦); potential camping	84.5	⬦ ▲
12.0	**MILE MARKER 12;** swampy area	84.4	
12.2	Large seasonal drainage	84.2	
12.7	ATV track at top of hill	83.7	

MILES W→E	TRAIL POINT	MILES E→W	NOTES
12.8	Creek (low volume, good water 🚰)	83.6	🚰
13.0	**MILE MARKER 13**	83.4	
13.1	Seasonal creek	83.3	
13.3	Pipeline right-of-way; gravel FS 204B	83.1	
13.7	Creek (stagnant water)	82.7	
14.0	**MILE MARKER 14**	82.4	
14.1	ATV track	82.3	
14.2	FS 271 (good dirt road); FS 204 (paved road); Kelly's Pond Hunter Camp 1 mi right on FS 271	82.2	▬ Ⓐ
14.6	ATV track	81.8	
15.0	**MILE MARKER 15**; potential camping; creek (low volume, murky 🚰)	81.4	🚰 ▲
15.5	Seasonal creek	80.9	
15.8	LSHT Stubblefield Trailhead Parking Lot 6, FM 1375	80.6	▬ 🅿
★ **SECTION 3**			
15.8	LSHT Stubblefield Trailhead Parking Lot 6, FM 1375	80.6	▬ 🅿
16.0	**MILE MARKER 16**	80.4	
16.5	Lake Conroe shoreline; ◊◊◊◊◊ large campsite	79.9	◊ ▲
16.8	Creek (medium volume; slow-flowing, semiclear water 🚰)	79.6	🚰
17.0	**MILE MARKER 17**	79.4	
17.3	Potential campsite	79.1	▲
17.6	Bridge over seasonal drainage; wetlands	78.8	
17.9	Bridge over Quicksand Creek (medium volume, good water ◊◊◊◊)	78.5	◊
18.0	Cross seasonal drainage; **MILE MARKER 18**	78.4	
18.3	FS 215B (closed to vehicles)	78.1	
19.0	**MILE MARKER 19**	77.4	
19.2	Swampy creek (stagnant water)	77.2	
19.7	Stubblefield Lake Campground	76.7	🚰 Ⓐ
20.0	FS 215/Stubblefield Lake Rd. bridge*; **MILE MARKER 20**	76.4	▬
20.3	End road walk, reenter woods to right of road	76.1	
21.0	**MILE MARKER 21**; Gus Randel Rd.; utilities right-of-way	75.4	▬

MILES W→E	TRAIL POINT	MILES E→W	NOTES
21.4	ATV track	75.0	
21.5	Potential campsites	74.9	▲
21.7	Fire break or pipeline right-of-way	74.7	
21.9	Seasonal creek	74.5	
22.0	**MILE MARKER 22;** property boundary	74.4	
22.2	Stony-bottomed seasonal creek	74.2	
22.3	Right on old jeep track	74.1	
22.6	Jeep road splits; take left fork	73.8	
23.0	Private farm on left; **MILE MARKER 23**	73.4	
23.1	FM 1374	73.3	✖
23.5	Left on large dirt road for a few hundred feet	72.9	
24.0	Fern Creek; ◊◊◊◊ **MILE MARKER 24**	72.4	◊
24.5	Right on dirt road for 0.2 mi	71.9	
24.7	Left on LSHT; reenter woods	71.7	
25.0	**MILE MARKER 25**	71.4	
25.2	Large seasonal drainage	71.2	
25.3	Old logging road	71.1	
26.0	**MILE MARKER 26**	70.4	
26.1	Right on jeep track	70.3	
26.4	Right on dirt Bath Road	70.0	✖
27.9	Intersection of Bath and Ball Roads; right on Ball Road	68.5	✖
28.1	Left on gravel Cotton Creek Cemetery Road	68.3	✖
28.3	National-forest property boundary; left on old dirt road	68.1	

The bridge at Mile Marker 20 (see previous page) is expected to reopen no sooner than August 2020.

★ SECTION 4

28.3	National-forest property boundary; left on old dirt road	68.1	
28.4	Leave old dirt road; right over hump into woods on LSHT	68.0	
28.9	Pond; ◊◊◊ designated camping	67.5	◊ ⓐ
29.0	**MILE MARKER 29**	67.4	
29.5	Seasonal drainage	66.9	
30.0	Cross pipeline right-of-way; **MILE MARKER 30**	66.4	

MILES W→E	TRAIL POINT	MILES E→W	NOTES
30.7	Enter open area with potential camping; seasonal drainage	65.7	▲
31.0	Seasonal drainage; **MILE MARKER 31**	65.4	
31.3	Elkins Lake water-treatment plant visible	65.1	
31.5	Seasonal stream	64.9	
32.0	**MILE MARKER 32;** Elkins Lake subdivision; left on paved road	64.4	☰
32.1	Cross Camelia Lake spillway (likely polluted)	64.3	
32.6	Seasonal drainage; potential waterless campsites in pine forest	63.8	▲
33.0	**MILE MARKER 33**	63.4	
33.1	Cross tributary of Alligator Branch; enter swamplands	63.3	
33.3	Alligator Branch (low flow, clear, spring-fed ◊◊◊◊)	63.1	◊ ▲
33.8	Cross old rail bed; shortcut 1.6 mi to Huntsville State Park to right	62.6	Ⓐ 🅿
34.0	**MILE MARKER 34**	62.4	
34.7	Junction of trails; right on LSHT	61.7	
35.0	**MILE MARKER 35;** I-45; LSHT Huntsville Trailhead Parking Lot 7; right on I-45 feeder road	61.4	☰ 🅿
35.6	Left on Park Road 40; continue under I-45 (Huntsville State Park is about 1 mile right on PR 40)	60.8	☰
36.6	Right on TX 75	59.8	☰
36.7	Left on Evelyn Lane	59.7	☰
36.9	Left on LSHT, to the right of blue metal gate	59.5	
★ SECTION 5			
36.9	Left into woods right of blue metal gate	59.5	☰
37.0	**MILE MARKER 37**	59.4	
37.4	Seasonal drainage; abandoned logging road	59.0	
37.6	Large, sandy-bottomed gully	58.8	
37.7	Steep-sided seasonal drainage	58.7	
37.8	Jeep track	58.6	
38.0	**MILE MARKER 38;** open, grassy area; potential campsite	58.4	▲

MILES W→E	TRAIL POINT	MILES E→W	NOTES
38.2	Bridge over small seasonal creek (stagnant water)	58.2	
38.3	Phelps Primitive Campsite	58.1	Ⓐ
38.4	Grass-covered logging road	58.0	
38.6	Old wooden milepost 38	57.8	
38.7	Seasonal drainage	57.7	
38.9	Potential campsite	57.5	▲
39.0	**MILE MARKER 39**	57.4	
39.1	Left on jeep track across power line	57.3	
39.3	Hiker gate; left onto gravel Evelyn Lane	57.1	▰
39.7	Reenter woods on left	56.7	
40.0	Old logging road; **MILE MARKER 40**	56.4	
40.4	Bridged seasonal creek (small amount of flowing water)	56.0	
40.5	Large seasonal creek (stagnant water)	55.9	
40.6	Seasonal creek	55.8	
41.0	**MILE MARKER 41**	55.4	
41.2	Gravel road	55.2	
41.6	Old logging road	54.8	
41.7	Seasonal drainage	54.7	
41.9	Pipeline crossing	54.5	
42.0	**MILE MARKER 42**; left on FM 2296	54.4	▰
42.6	Right on Four Notch Road	53.8	▰
42.8	Cross railroad tracks; continue on Four Notch Road	53.6	
43.0	Creek (low volume 🚰); **MILE MARKER 43** along Four Notch Road	53.4	🚰
43.7	Cross Winters Bayou (high volume 🚰) on Four Notch Road bridge (*note:* pastures nearby)	52.7	🚰
44.0	**MILE MARKER 44**; Four Notch Road	52.4	
44.9	Left on dirt FS 213	51.5	▰
45.0	**MILE MARKER 45**, FS 213	51.4	
45.1	LSHT Four Notch Trailhead Parking Lot 8; reenter woods on right	51.3	▰ 🅿 Ⓐ

MILES W→E	TRAIL POINT	MILES E→W	NOTES
★ **SECTION 6**			
45.1	LSHT Four Notch Trailhead Parking Lot 8; Four Notch Hunter Camp; reenter woods on right	51.3	⛔ 🅿 ⓐ
45.4	Junction with Four Notch Loop Trail (red-blazed); main LSHT turns right	51.0	
45.7	Deep seasonal drainage; logging road	50.7	
45.9	Seasonal creek	50.5	
46.0	Faint logging road; **MILE MARKER 46**	50.4	
46.2	Seasonal creek	50.2	
46.5	Hunter camp on dirt FS 223; potential campsites	49.9	▲
46.7	Potential camping on right; parallel seasonal drainage on right	49.7	▲
46.8	Large seasonal creek	49.6	
47.0	**MILE MARKER 47**; seasonal creek 💧💧	49.4	💧
47.1	Left on old logging road	49.3	
47.2	Cross logging road	49.2	
47.4	Large, open flat; potential camping	49.0	▲
47.5	Right on old logging road	48.9	
47.6	Large, open flat; potential camping; seasonal creek 💧	48.8	💧 ▲
47.8	Junction of old logging roads	48.6	
48.0	**MILE MARKER 48**	48.4	
48.2	Boswell Creek (high volume, good water 💧💧💧💧); camping	48.2	💧 ▲
48.7	Seasonal drainage	47.7	
49.0	**MILE MARKER 49**	47.4	
49.4	Junction with Four Notch Loop Trail (red-blazed)	47.0	
49.5	Small seasonal drainage; hill	46.9	
49.7	Briar Creek (low flow, good water 🚰)	46.7	🚰
50.0	**MILE MARKER 50**	46.4	
50.4	Cross FS 206	46.0	⛔
51.0	**MILE MARKER 51**; pipeline right-of-way	45.4	
51.1	Large, seasonal Brandy Creek 💧	45.3	💧

MILES W→E	TRAIL POINT	MILES E→W	NOTES
51.4	Karolyi Primitive Campsite	45.0	Ⓐ
51.5	Pond on left (dark, tannin-colored water ◊◊◊); camping	44.9	◊ ▲
51.7	Left on gravel FS 200 (no parking)	44.7	▭▭
51.9	Creek (low volume, good water 🚰) along FS 200	44.5	🚰
52.4	Right on gravel FS 207 at stop sign	44.0	▭▭
53.0	Gas-processing plant	43.4	
54.4	Junction of FS 207 and 202; reenter woods	42.0	▭▭ 🅿
★ SECTION 7			
54.4	Junction of FS 207 and 202; reenter woods	42.0	▭▭ 🅿
54.6	Deep seasonal drainage; potential camping	41.8	▲
55.0	Series of seasonal drainages; **MILE MARKER 55**	41.4	
55.3	Twin seasonal drainages	41.1	
55.4	Cross sunken road twice; potential camping	41.0	▲
55.8	Cross seasonal drainage twice (stagnant water)	40.6	
56.0	**MILE MARKER 56;** cross drainage to the left in 0.1 mi	40.4	
56.2	Seasonal drainage; West Fork Caney Creek (trickle of water)	40.2	
56.9	West Fork Caney Creek (low volume, clear water 🚰); property boundary	39.5	🚰
57.0	**MILE MARKER 57**	39.4	
57.7	Shallow seasonal drainage; larger U-shaped drainage	38.7	
58.0	**MILE MARKER 58;** potential camping	38.4	▲
58.1	Old road bed	38.3	
58.2	Cross fern-lined seasonal drainage twice	38.2	
58.5	Signed 0.1-mi side trail to FS 202	37.9	
58.6	Pond off-trail 50 yd left; ◊◊◊◊ potential camping	37.8	◊ ▲
58.8	Large oak tree; potential camping	37.6	▲
59.0	**MILE MARKER 59**	37.4	
59.1	Fern-lined Chinquapin Creek; potential camping	37.3	▲
59.5	Seasonal drainage	36.9	
59.8	Primitive campsite; FS 202D (closed to vehicles)	36.6	Ⓐ

MILES W→E	TRAIL POINT	MILES E→W	NOTES
60.0	**MILE MARKER 60;** several small drainages and old logging road	36.4	
60.2	Old jeep track heads uphill to left; follow LSHT straight ahead	36.2	
60.4	Cross large, sandy-bottomed intermittent stream	36.0	
60.6	Cross several small seasonal drainages	35.8	
60.9	Junction of trails; follow LSHT left	35.5	
61.0	**MILE MARKER 61**	35.4	
61.4	Open area at junction of logging roads; potential camping; follow LSHT straight and then right	35.0	▲
61.5	Make a sharp left turn	34.9	
61.7	Deep, brushy, seasonal drainage	34.7	
62.0	**MILE MARKER 62**	34.4	
62.4	Fencepost and corner at property boundary	34.0	
62.5	Potential camping left of trail	33.9	▲
62.8	LSHT Big Woods Trailhead Parking Lot 9; follow LSHT left onto dirt Ira Denson Rd.	33.6	⛐ 🅿
★ SECTION 8			
62.8	LSHT Big Woods Trailhead Parking Lot 9; follow LSHT left on dirt Ira Denson Rd.	33.6	⛐ 🅿
63.0	Intersection of Ira Denson Rd. and FS 202	33.4	⛐
64.7	Intersection of FS 202/John Warren Rd. and TX 150; follow LSHT left on TX 150	31.7	⛐
65.0	Intersection of TX 150 and FM 945 in Evergreen; Evergreen Baptist Church (water 🚰); follow LSHT right on FM 945	31.4	⛐ 🚰
65.5	Cemetery on left along FM 945	30.9	
67.4	Intersection of FM 945 and Butch Arthur Rd. (Jacobs Rd.); LSHT Trailhead Parking Lot 10	29.0	⛐ 🅿
67.9	Seasonal drainage	28.5	
68.0	**MILE MARKER 68**	28.4	
68.2	Hiker bridge over large seasonal drainage (low flow, good water 🚰)	28.2	🚰
68.4	Seasonal drainage	28.0	

MILES W→E	TRAIL POINT	MILES E→W	NOTES
68.6	LSHT Primitive Campsite 2, to right of trail	27.8	Ⓐ
69.0	**MILE MARKER 69**	27.4	
69.1	Fence corner	27.3	
69.2	Creek (low flow, good water 🚰)	27.2	🚰
69.3	Fence corner	27.1	
69.4	Creek (low flow, good water 🚰)	27.0	🚰
69.8	ATV track; horse farm	26.6	
69.9	Freeside Ln. (dirt road)	26.5	
70.0	**MILE MARKER 70**	26.4	
70.1	Hiker bridge over drainage (low flow, good water 🚰)	26.3	🚰
70.6	Hiker gate; stay straight	25.8	
71.0	**MILE MARKER 70;** straight on LSHT	25.4	
71.1	East Fork of the San Jacinto River 🌢🌢🌢🌢🌢	25.3	🌢
71.3	Hiker bridge over creek (deep, clear water 🚰)	25.1	🚰
71.6	Hiker bridge over stream (shallow, clear water 🚰)	24.8	🚰
72.0	**MILE MARKER 72;** pipeline right-of-way; gravel jeep track	24.4	
72.2	Hiker bridge over creek (shallow, clear water 🌢🌢🌢🌢)	24.2	🌢
72.3	Potential campsite on left	24.1	▲
72.4	Gravel road (FS 280D); utilities right-of-way	24.0	
72.6	Old logging road	23.8	
72.8	Gas-pipeline service road	23.6	
72.9	FS 280B (closed)	23.5	
73.0	**MILE MARKER 73**	23.4	
73.1	Sharp right turn; hiker bridge over seasonal drainage	23.3	
73.7	FM 2025; LSHT Iron Ore Trailhead Parking Lot 11	22.7	▬ 🅿
73.8	Potential camping close to road; utility lines	22.6	▲
73.9	Side trail to LSHT Parking Lot 11	22.5	
74.0	**MILE MARKER 74**	22.4	
74.8	Mountain bike trail	21.6	
74.9	Mountain bike trail	21.5	

MILES W→E	TRAIL POINT	MILES E→W	NOTES
75.0	Double Lake Recreation Area; **MILE MARKER 75**	21.4	⚊ 🚰 Ⓐ 🅿
★ **SECTION 9**			
75.0	Double Lake Recreation Area; **MILE MARKER 75**	21.4	⚊ 🚰 Ⓐ 🅿
75.1	Utilities right-of-way; intersect mountain bike trail	21.3	
75.6	Gravel FS 220; hiker gate; Double Lake Branch (good water, medium flow 〇〇〇) on left	20.8	⚊ ◊
75.7	Hiker bridge over seasonal drainage; LSHT Primitive Campsite 1	20.7	Ⓐ
76.0	Small bridge over deep drainage; potential camping; creek on left (good water, low flow); **MILE MARKER 76**	20.4	🚰 ▲
76.4	Small bridge over deep drainage	20.0	
76.6	Ford wide creek (bridge destroyed in 2017; low flow, good water 🚰)	19.8	🚰
76.9	Two bridges over small creeks (low flow, good water 🚰)	19.5	🚰
77.0	**MILE MARKER 77**	19.4	
77.6	Cross swampy creek (stagnant water)	18.8	
78.0	**MILE MARKER 78**	18.4	
78.1	Picnic spot off LSHT along banks of Double Lake Branch	18.3	
78.6	Cross old rail bed; left on LSHT	17.8	
79.0	**MILE MARKER 79**	17.4	
79.2	Intersect orange-blazed Big Creek Trail; left on LSHT	17.2	
79.3	Intersect green-blazed White Oak Trail; left on LSHT	17.1	
79.4	Bridge over Big Creek (high flow, good water 〇〇〇〇〇)	17.0	◊
79.7	Long bridge over Big Creek; intersect yellow-blazed Pine Trail; left on LSHT	16.7	◊
79.8	Hiker bridge; intersect trail heading down to left; sharp right on LSHT	16.6	
79.9	BIG CREEK SCENIC AREA sign; short side trail to left leads to LSHT Trailhead Parking Lot 12; intersect yellow-blazed Pine Trail and orange-blazed Big Creek Trail on right; straight on LSHT on old rail bed	16.5	🅿
80.0	**MILE MARKER 80**	16.4	
80.6	Bench; potential waterless camp	15.8	▲

MILES W→E	TRAIL POINT	MILES E→W	NOTES
80.9	FS 221	15.5	▭
81.0	**MILE MARKER 81;** potential waterless camp	15.4	▲
81.2	Intersect unidentified trail; left on LSHT; potential campsite; seasonal drainage	15.2	▲
81.5	Upper reaches of Tarkington Bayou (seasonal flow, good water 🚰)	14.9	🚰
82.0	**MILE MARKER 82**	14.4	
82.5	LSHT Tarkington Trailhead Parking Lot 13; FM 2666	13.9	▭ 🅿

★ SECTION 10

MILES W→E	TRAIL POINT	MILES E→W	NOTES
82.5	LSHT Trailhead Parking Lot 13; FM 2666	13.9	▭ 🅿
83.0	**MILE MARKER 83**	13.4	
83.5	Corner benchmark and bearing tree; 0.6-mi side trail to designated campsite	12.9	Ⓐ
83.6	Designated campsite	12.8	Ⓐ
83.7	Bridge over creek (stagnant water)	12.7	
84.0	**MILE MARKER 84;** seasonal drainage	12.4	
84.3	Reach banks of Tarkington Bayou ◊	12.1	◊
84.6	Hiker bridge over seasonal creek 🚰	11.8	🚰
84.9	Potential campsite	11.5	▲
85.0	**MILE MARKER 85;** pond ◊◊◊ 50 yd east; pipeline and access road	11.4	◊
86.0	**MILE MARKER 86**	10.4	
86.2	Old logging road; follow LSHT left, then right	10.2	
86.4	Oxbow pond of Tarkington Bayou (muddy) ◊◊◊	10.0	◊
87.0	**MILE MARKER 87**	9.4	
87.6	Veer away from Tarkington Bayou for good	8.8	
88.0	**MILE MARKER 88**	8.4	
88.3	Pipeline right-of-way	8.1	
88.7	Seasonal drainage	7.7	
89.0	**MILE MARKER 89;** left on logging road; Mercy Primitive Campsite	7.4	Ⓐ
89.3	Sharp turn to right	7.1	

MILES W→E	TRAIL POINT	MILES E→W	NOTES
90.0	**MILE MARKER 90**; semipaved Forest Valley Dr. near private homes	6.4	▅▅
90.1	Abandoned jeep roads; confusing junction; follow LSHT slightly to right and then straight	6.3	
90.2	Potential waterless campsite	6.2	▲
90.9	FM 2025; LSHT Trailhead Parking Lot 14 (store 0.9 mi south)	5.5	▅▅ 🅿
★ **SECTION 11**			
90.9	FM 2025; LSHT Trailhead Parking Lot 14 (store 0.9 mi south)	5.5	▅▅ 🅿
91.0	**MILE MARKER 91**	5.4	
91.2	Potential camping	5.2	▲
91.4	Cross at junction of small creeks (low flow, clear water, unreliable 🚰)	5.0	🚰
91.6	Right on old rail bed	4.8	
92.0	Unbridged seasonal creek (strong flow, clear water 🚰); **MILE MARKER 92**	4.4	🚰
92.6	Steel hiker bridge over East Fork of the San Jacinto River (deep, muddy water) ◊◊◊◊◊	3.8	◊
92.7	Seasonal creek (stagnant water)	3.7	
93.0	**MILE MARKER 93**; bridge over wetland	3.4	
93.1	TX 945 (store 1.3 mi east)	3.3	▅▅
93.4	Old fire-tower base	3.0	
93.8	Creek; ◊ small pond on right (north)	2.6	◊
94.0	Creek (clear water, good flow 🚰); **MILE MARKER 94**; old fire-tower base	2.4	🚰
94.5	Old fire-tower base	1.9	
94.7	Gravel FS 274A	1.7	
95.0	**MILE MARKER 95**; pipeline with road; hiker bridge over seasonal creek	1.4	
95.2	Boardwalk over palmetto swamp	1.2	
95.8	Steel hiker bridge over Winters Bayou (deep, muddy water) ◊◊◊◊◊	0.6	◊
95.9	Phone lines; boardwalk over wet area	0.5	
96.0	**MILE MARKER 96**	0.4	

MILES W→E	TRAIL POINT	MILES E→W	NOTES
96.1	Bridge over shallow drainage	0.3	
96.4	LSHT Trailhead Parking Lot 15; FM 1725; eastern terminus of LSHT	0.0	⚏ 🅿

MILEAGE CHART KEY

▲	Undeveloped campsite or potential camping area	🚰	Water source (seasonal/unrated)
Ⓐ	Designated campsite during hunting season	⚏	Major roads (jeep tracks and logging roads are not indicated)
🜄	Water source (DROPS-rated)	🅿	Parking area/trailhead

A still life of tree lichen and ferns in Big Creek Scenic Area

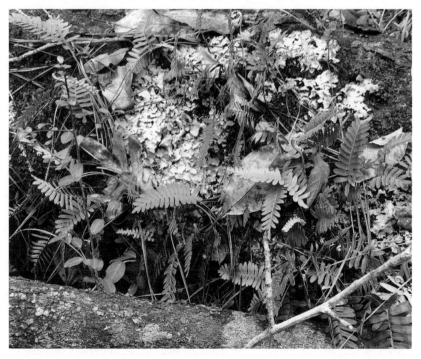

ACKNOWLEDGMENTS

I WOULD NEVER HAVE followed my calling to further explore and document the Lone Star Hiking Trail (LSHT) without the steady encouragement and support of my partner on trails and in life, Andy Somers. Andy also created and later edited all of the maps in this guidebook—an enormous undertaking that I could not have accomplished on my own.

During my original thru-hike of the LSHT as I collected data for this guidebook, I had the assistance and good company of Debbie Richardson Waizenegger. She helped me push the measuring wheel and kept me honest regarding right and left.

My second attempt at thru-hiking ended abruptly due to rough weather, later requiring multiple forays and day hikes during limited time off from real life, so I'm greatly indebted to my family's patience and, at times, on-ground assistance. My husband and daughter, Maddie, spent several days hiking and collecting data with me, and they kept me going when the weather and time constraints seemed always stacked against me.

My father, James Borski, drove me to and from the trail on many occasions and always provided a comfortable base of operations. Not only that, but my dad instilled in me a love of the outdoors and of all the landscapes of Texas.

Brandt Mannchen of the Lone Star Chapter of the Sierra Club and Bill Anderson of the U.S. Forest Service were exceptionally generous with their time and information about the trail and its history.

On his own thru-hike, Bill Sadd of Fredericksburg, Texas, voluntarily kept a detailed account of trail features while utilizing this guidebook, sending me an extremely detailed set of notes and updates that served as an independent field test, solidifying and improving the guide.

Dave Wade gave me permission to borrow his DROPS water-availability system, which he created for use by the Lone Star Hiking Trail Club (LSHTC).

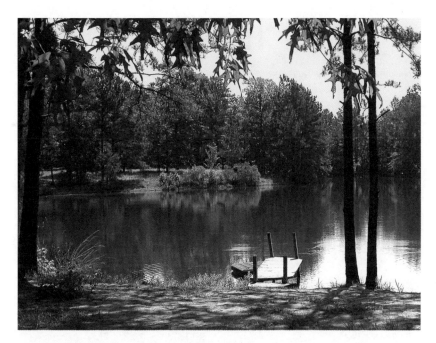

Neiderhofer Lake, a short hike off the LSHT in Section 6, is a peaceful and secluded diversion.   Photo: Jeff Stull

June Aaron, Jeff Borski, James Borski, Roslyn Bullas, Ritchey Halphen, Tim Jackson, Steve Jones, Brandt Mannchen, Scott McGrew, Molly Merkle, Cathy Murphy, Laura Shauger, Andy Somers, Dave Wade, and Linda Woolf all provided much-needed advice and assistance with enhancing and editing both editions of the book. To everyone who gave freely of their care and time, I am greatly indebted.

A special thanks to Evergreen Baptist Church for allowing hikers to use their water taps as they walk through the hamlet of Evergreen, Texas.

I must also express my personal gratitude to the many volunteers who built and still maintain the LSHT, beginning with the trail's inception by Orrin Bonney and the many other volunteers from the Lone Star Chapter of the Sierra Club whose dedication and muscle mapped and carved the trail through the thick woods in 1960s and '70s—without them the trail would not exist.

A portion of the proceeds from the sale of this book will be donated to the Lone Star Chapter of the Sierra Club and the LSHTC, nonprofit organizations that continue to protect and promote the trail.

INDEX

ABOUT THE AUTHOR

KAREN BORSKI SOMERS is a native of Spring, Texas. She studied biomedical engineering at Texas A&M University and has spent most of her career working for NASA contractors in Clear Lake, Texas, and Huntsville, Alabama. In 1998 she thru-hiked the 2,165-mile Appalachian Trail solo, and in 2004 she hiked the 2,650-mile Pacific Crest Trail with her husband, Andy. Karen's trail name is *Nocona,* a Comanche word meaning "the wanderer." She has hiked and backpacked in 36 US states, logging more than 9,000 trail miles. She also bicycled 4,400 miles across the US, from the Atlantic to the Pacific, on the TransAmerica Bicycle Trail in 2005. Karen currently resides with her husband, two daughters, and their hiking Sheltie in northern Alabama. They continue to wander on and off trails.

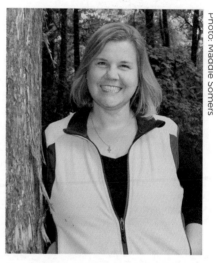

Photo: Maddie Somers